HEALTH EDUCATION: THE SEARCH FOR VALUES

DONALD A. READ
WORCESTER STATE COLLEGE

SIDNEY B. SIMON
UNIVERSITY OF MASSACHUSETTS

JOEL B. GOODMAN
NATIONAL HUMANISTIC EDUCATION CENTER

HEALTH EDUCATION: THE SEARCH FOR VALUES

PRENTICE-HALL, INC.
ENGLEWOOD CLIFFS, NEW JERSEY 07632

Library of Congress Cataloging in Publication Data

READ, DONALD A
   Health education.

   Bibliography: p.
   Includes index.
   1. Health education. 2. Moral education.
3. Values. I. Simon, Sidney B., (date) joint author. II. Goodman, Joel B., (date) joint author. III. Title. [DNLM: 1. Health education. WA590 R279h]
RA440.R43   613'.07'1   76-54148
ISBN 0-13-384511-7

HEALTH EDUCATION: THE SEARCH FOR VALUES

Donald A. Read, Sidney B. Simon, and Joel B. Goodman

© 1977 by Prentice-Hall, Inc., Englewood Cliffs, N.J. 07632

All rights reserved.
No part of this book may be reproduced in any form
or by any means
without permission in writing from the publisher.

Printed in the United States of America
10 9 8 7 6 5 4 3 2 1

          Prentice-Hall International, Inc., *London*
          Prentice-Hall of Australia Pty. Limited, *Sydney*
          Prentice-Hall of Canada, Ltd., *Toronto*
          Prentice-Hall of India Private Limited, *New Delhi*
          Prentice-Hall of Japan, Inc., *Tokyo*
          Prentice-Hall of Southeast Asia Pte. Ltd., *Singapore*
          Whitehall Books Limited, *Wellington, New Zealand*

This book is dedicated to:

Wesley W. Staton
who gave me direction

Louis E. Raths
a most important teacher in my life.

Yetta Cohen
a grandma for all seasons

CONTENTS

Preface *ix*

1 **ABOUT TEACHING** *1*
The Evidence Suggests A Need for Change *1*
Ways of Effecting Change *3*
Our Hope As You Move On In This Book *5*

2 **ABOUT VALUES CLARIFICATION** *7*
Values, Values Everywhere . . . *7*
Values Clarification: In the Beginning *8*
What's Everybody Running For? . . . The Need for Values Clarification *10*
Values Clarification: A Nutshell Summary *16*

3 **1 + 1 = 3:**
VALUES CLARIFICATION + HEALTH EDUCATION *19*
The Dynamic Duo *19*
Values Clarification: Moving from Health Information to Health Education *21*
Values Clarification and Health Education: Where and How *23*
A Summary *33*

vii

4 **VALUES CLARIFICATION ACTIVITIES: A TASTE FOR SOME BREAD-AND-BUTTER STRATEGIES** *35*

The Purpose of the Activities *36*
The Context of the Activities *36*
Directions for the Activities *37*
Strategies in Human Sexuality *40*
Strategies in Drug Education *60*
Strategies in Nutrition Education *74*

5 **WRITING ACTIVITIES** *87*

The Personal Diary *87*
Strategies in Human Sexuality *88*
Strategies in Drug Education *95*
Strategies in Nutrition Education *98*

6 **WORKING THROUGH AN EXERCISE** *101*

Stepping Back For A Minute *102*

7 **PROCESSING** *107*

Exercise: Name Tags *108*
Exercise: Emergency Now *113*

8 **A HUMANISTIC APPROACH TO EVALUATION AND WAYS OF EVALUATING HUMANISTIC EDUCATION: COUNTING THE APPLES IN A SEED** *121*

Guidelines for Humanistic Evaluation *122*
Evaluation Activities: A Baker's Dozen *126*
A Quick Summary and a Request for Feedback *138*

9 **A FINAL NOTE** *141*

Summary *145*

APPENDICES *147*

Terminology *147*
References *155*
Additional Value Sheets: A Sampling *156*
Films in Values Clarification *166*
Tapes and Cassettes in Values Clarification *169*
A Review of Books in Values Clarification *170*
Additional Readings to Grow On *177*
Materials Available from the National Humanistic Education Center *181*

INDEX *183*

PREFACE

Should I smoke? How do my personal values influence my level of health? Am I a significant person? Are my values my own? How can I improve my life? Love—how much do I need? Should I get married now? What do I think about myself? Is my life meaningful? How can I change my life?

Health Education: The Search for Values helps teachers (and students) to deal with these and related questions in the classroom, in a counseling situation, in small groups. It offers, for the first time under one cover, theory, guidelines, approaches, and tools in values clarification as it applies to the area of health.

Values clarification, upon which *Health Education: The Search for Values* is based, follows up on tne pioneering work of Louis Raths, Merrill Harmin, and Sidney B. Simon, who first offered values clarification as a coherent model in their book *Values and Teaching,* which is in turn based on the work of John Dewey.

Values clarification represents one branch of humanistic education and is concerned with the process of *valuing—how* values originate and *how* they may be changed—rather than on the inculcation of one particular set of values. Through the values-clarification approach, students can develop value-able skills (how to's) in the cognitive, affective, active, and interpersonal realms.

One of our values is that these skills are at least as important as (but not mutually exclusive of) the "basic skills" (the 3 R's). In fact, they are life-long, basic, human living skills. And so, we strongly urge teachers, counselors, parents, nurses, and other helping professionals to become familiar with this approach, in addition to taking courses on methods and materials in sociology, psychology, science and social studies.

Health Education: The Search for Values is meant to be a nourishing book and an alive one—a book in which the reader can carry on a dialogue with the authors. This book offers a smorgasbord of food for thought on such topics as the history, guidelines, and skills involved in values clarification; ways of integrating values clarification into health education; a wealth of examples of practical classroom activities that operationalize the theory and guidelines; thoughts on how to work through and process a values-clarification activity; humanistic methodology for evaluating values clarification; and a glossary of terms often used in this field. The appendices also include excellent sources/resources (e.g. films, books, tapes) for those who would like to pursue their interest in this area.

Our hope is that this book will be both a mirror and a springboard—a mirror for you, the reader, to focus on your own value (worth, ideas, wisdom) and your values (in health-related areas); and a springboard for using the ideas (from yourself and this book) in your own life and work. There is a great deal of joy and excitement awaiting you . . . the joy and excitement of learning something new about yourself, the joy and excitement of seeing one of your students discovering something new about him/herself, the joy and excitement of growing from the wisdom of your students.

In fact, the focus of this book could be summed up well by the comment of fifth-grader Sybil Behrens: "Love is knowing you have a reason for living." We intend to share with you ways of clarifying your reasons and your students' reasons—and ways to celebrate each and every person as value-able.

This book can be used in many varied ways. For example:

- It could become a course outline for a class on "Values Clarification in Health Education."

- It could be used as a basic text or supplemental text for a methods course in health education.

- It could be a valuable tool for those teachers "out in the field" who wish to try something new and exciting in their teaching.

- It could be used in any course in teaching, education, sociology, or psychology, as a guide to values clarification.

- Finally, this is a book of tools . . . tools to be used in creating a classroom atmosphere in which personal values become an important and vital aspect of the teaching-learning process.

We are serious about wishing this book to create a dialogue between authors and readers. At several points in the text we invite you, the reader, to communicate with us (see chapter 8 on evaluation). Your feedback, ideas (e.g. those generated on the worksheets in the chapter on bread-and-butter strategies), and questions are all welcomed. Also, if you want information on other values-clarification workshops and materials, please communicate with us through the National Humanistic Education Center, 110 Spring Street, Saratoga Springs, New York 12866, to the attention of Joel Goodman.

Ultimately, we hope this book will *make a difference*—to you and to your students. We extend our best wishes and support to you in your *search for values*.

Donald A. Read
Sidney B. Simon
Joel B. Goodman

P.S. With special appreciation to our Production Editor, Barbara Kanski, and to the Designer, Ben Kann, who have treated the book with TLC.

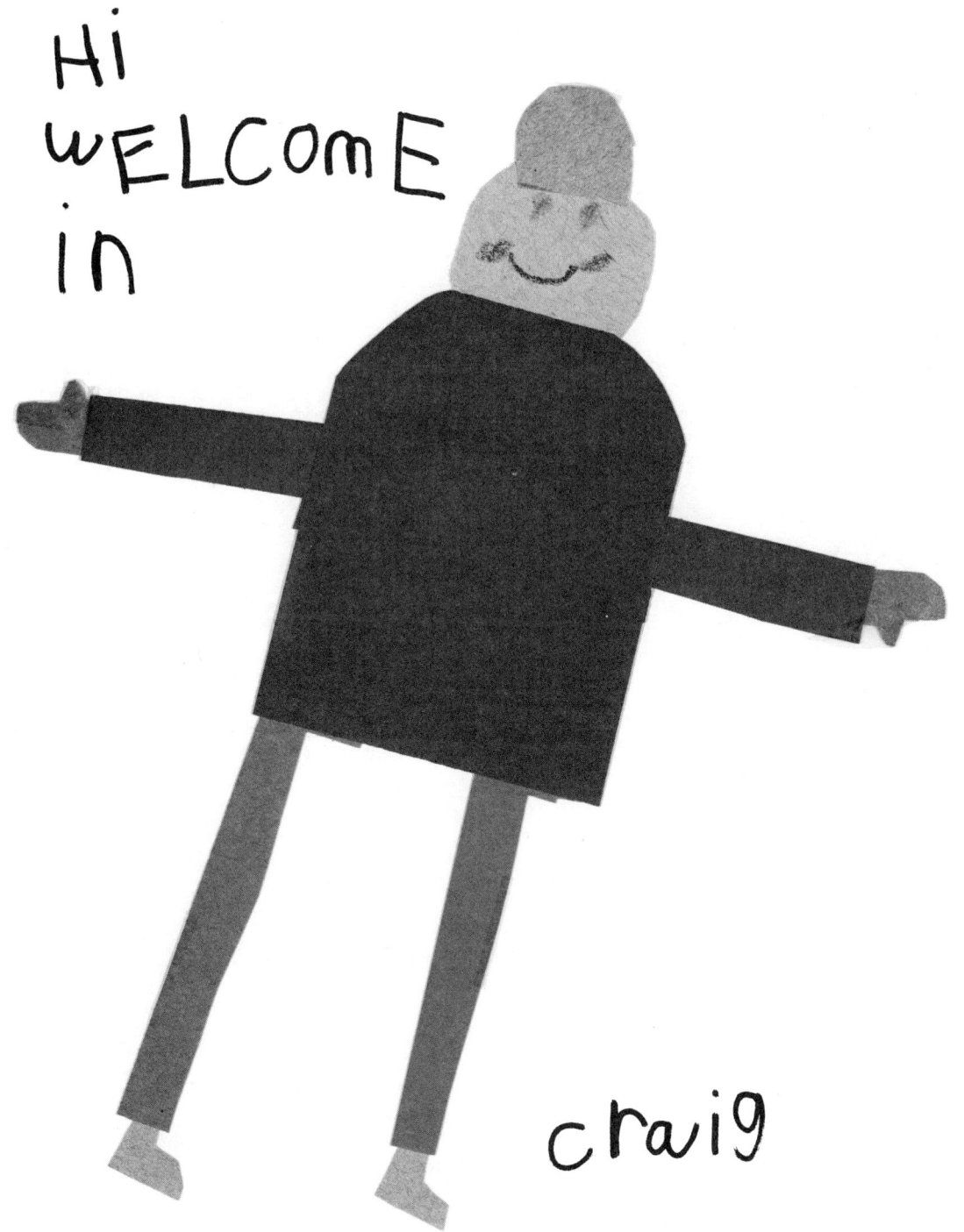

HEALTH EDUCATION: THE SEARCH FOR VALUES

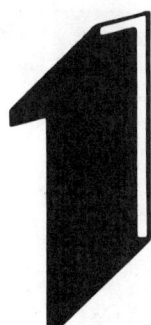

ABOUT TEACHING

Teacher: Why do you use drugs?
Student: Why not?
Teacher: Well, they are dangerous! How could I convince you to stop?
Student: Well, you could start by showing me something better.

This brief imaginary conversation may just contain the key to effective teaching in health—and that is that teaching facts alone is relatively ineffectual in changing health habits. And, as with other academic subjects, the goal of health education is to bring about positive changes in attitudes and behavior.

THE EVIDENCE SUGGESTS A NEED FOR CHANGE

We do not wish to downgrade the value of accurate information. Such information about health is necessary in the decision-making process. But, in and of itself, supplying accurate information is simply not enough, as recent evidence is beginning to show.

A panel established to review the drug education laws in New York State states that, "It is not a lack of information that leads young people to turn to drugs and alcohol." On the contrary, much instruction about drugs "stimulates unnecessary interest in the subject matter and may promote experimentation." (Legislature to Repeal Drug Education Laws, 1973.)

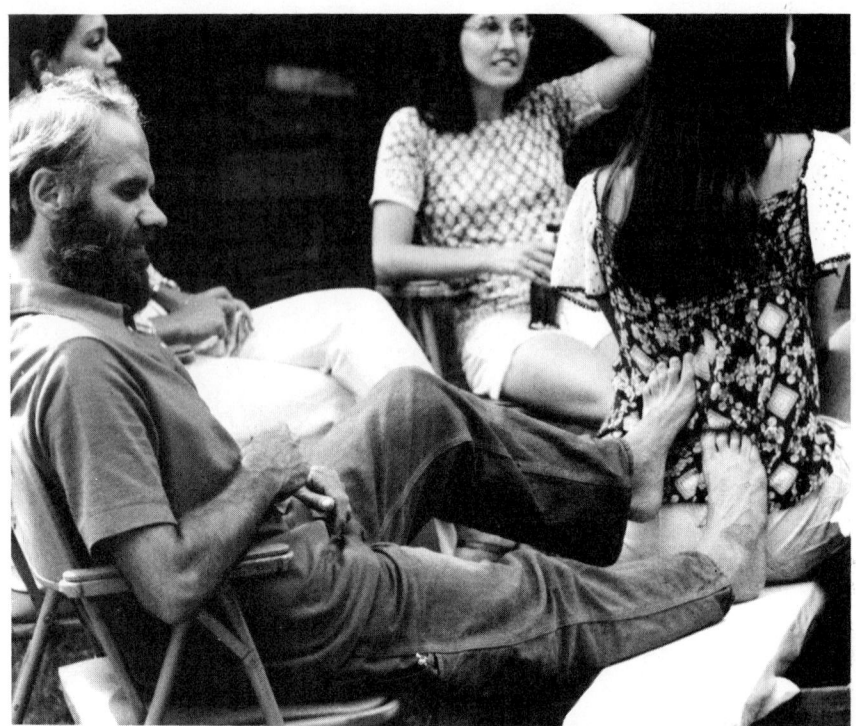

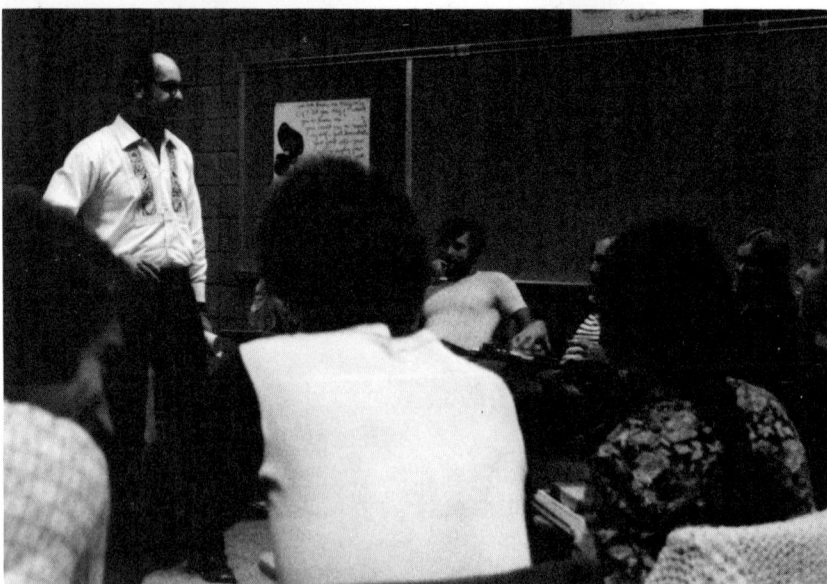

Learning to grow, being yourself, being and becoming what you want to become, becoming that person you value and love, may be the only person you will ultimately learn to love and grow with. (Don Read)

Dr. Herbert C. Modlin, Director of the Department of Preventive Psychiatry of the Menninger Foundation, in talking about society's reaction to drugs stated that, "there is no evidence that education prevented any drug usage, but some evidence that, after a course on drugs, the incidence of usage increased among the students." (Modlin, 1974.)

In the area of human sexuality, Dr. Karem J. Monsour, Director of the Counseling Center at the Clarement Colleges, has found that sex education courses and birth control information appear to be relatively ineffective in helping young women enter their own sexual lives with personal acceptance, understanding of their sexuality, and rational use of contraceptives. "Young women simply do not deal openly with sex in their own lives when they have been trained in a conspiracy of silence about it," he says. (Monsour, 1973.)

WAYS OF EFFECTING CHANGE

As we have stated before, we do not wish to downgrade the real value of accurate information, for such information can be a significant help in the decision-making process. But the real promise in health education (and *all* education, for that matter) is to engage the teacher in more actively working with self-image, communication skills, values, and decision-making skills in the classroom. This would also include helping students to make connections between the public knowledge—that is, the subject matter—that they are studying and their own private, personal concerns.

A number of writers have suggested ways in which we may be able to effect change. Among these are Mario D. Fantini and Gerald Weinstein, who propose that, "it seems more helpful to show teachers how to recognize concerns of pupils, and match content and procedures to these concerns, than it is to talk to them about love and understanding." (Fantini and Weinstein, 1968.)

Weinstein and Fantini defined three broad areas of student concerns: (1) "self-identity," which is the question of "Who am I?"; (2) "relationship," which is the quesion of "Who am I in relation to others? What's the quantity and quality of my relationships with others?"; and (3) the concerns for power, control, influence—"To what degree do I have control over what's happening in my own life?"

William Glasser, in his book *Schools Without Failure,* suggests that positive self-images of the unsure can be enhanced through positive approaches by teachers, open-ended class discussions with no "right" answers, and greater opportunity for decision-making by students. (Glasser, 1969.)

Happiness Is . . .

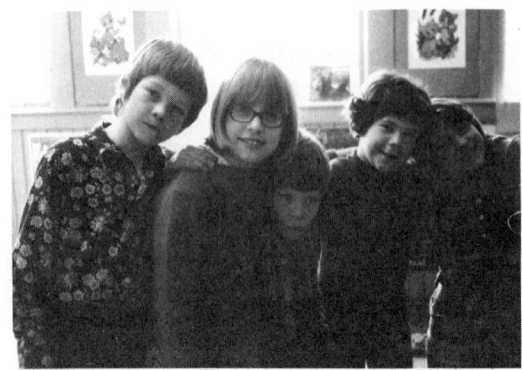
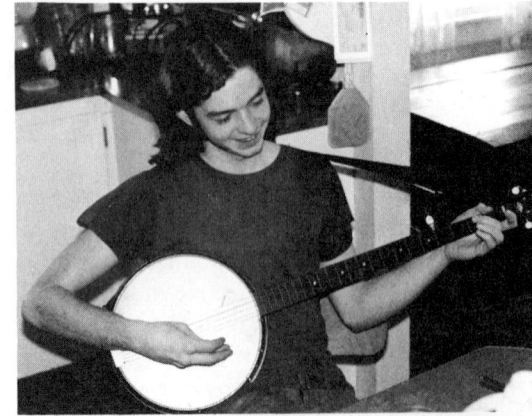
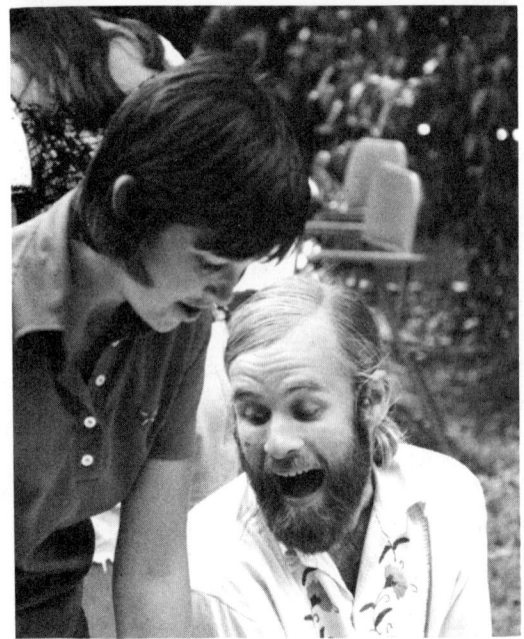
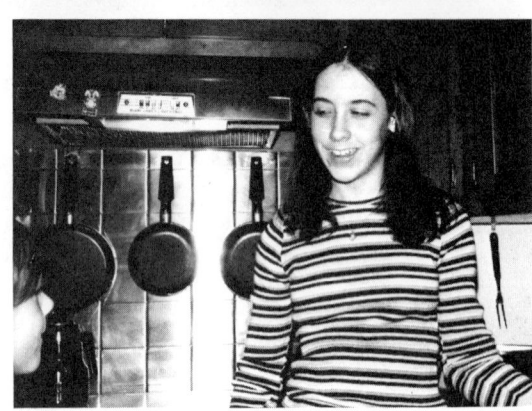

5 ABOUT TEACHING Chapter 1

Carl Rogers sees the perception of self as an untapped source of information for the teaching-learning environment. He states: "A person learns significantly only those things which he perceives as being involved in the maintenance of, or enhancement of, the structure of self."

OUR HOPE AS YOU MOVE ON IN THIS BOOK

Almost invariably, if the teacher's influence has been good, what the student remembers was the attention that was paid *him,* the respect his teacher accorded him, rather than the factual information that was taught.

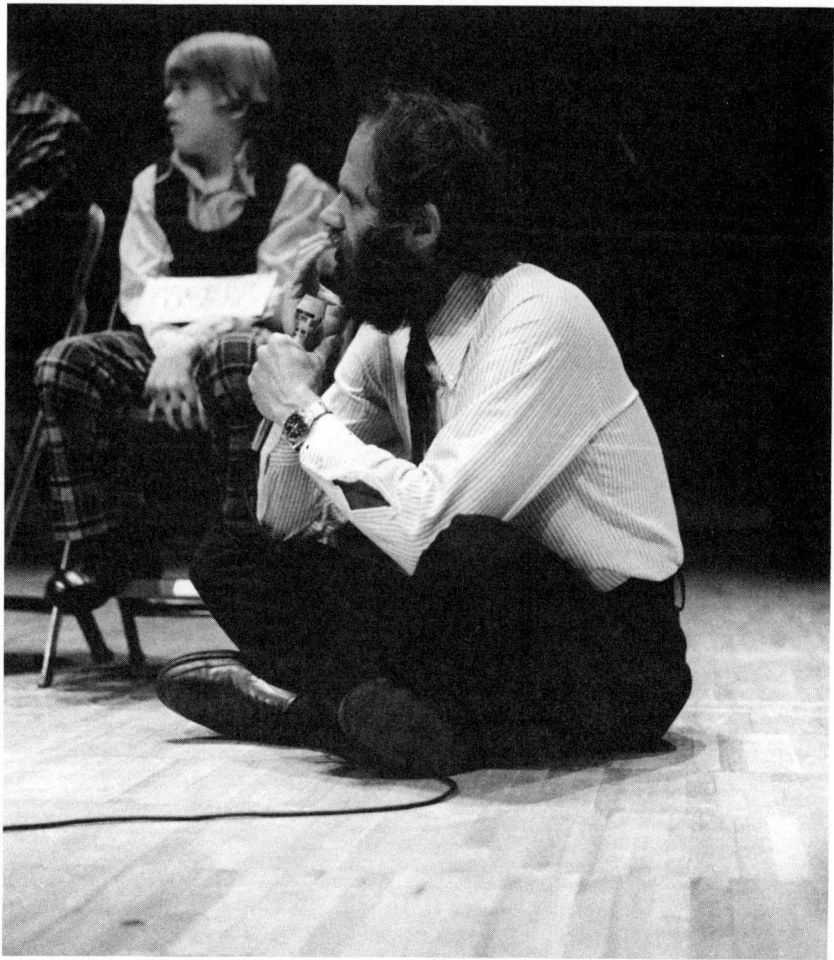

The real promise for bringing about effective health education lies in our ability to build positive images and strong feelings of self-worth in students by helping them to gain greater insights into their own value systems and develop their decision-making processes. This will require an ability on the part of the teacher to listen to students, tune in on their feelings, and allow and encourage them to open up so that they can express those feelings.

We hope that every good teacher labors daily toward this important end. At their best, teachers know well the things their credentials imply they have learned. But more than that, the good teacher loves his/her students—as far as human nature will allow—and has high respect for what they value. He or she exudes enthusiasm and love, yet never presumes to teach these qualities. In a warm, accepting, integrated classroom, where each member is loved for himself or herself intrinsically, where each student gives and takes according to what he or she is capable of, the teacher often finds the emphasis more and more focusing on the full and free development of students who are the fullest, most real, happiest people they can become.

REFERENCES

State of New York, *Anomalies in Drug Abuse Treatment.* Legislative Document no. 11, 1975.

Glasser, William. *Schools Without Failure.* New York: Harper & Row, 1969, p. xi.

Modlin, Herbert C. "One Psychiatrist Views Society's Reaction to Drugs: Inappropriate and Irrational." *National Observer,* 9 November 1974, p. 13-B.

Monsour, Karem J. "Openness About Sexuality Best Way to Avert Pregnancies." *American Journal of Orthopsychiatry* 43 (1973):804-14.

Weinstein, Gerald, and Fantini, Mario. *A Model for Developing Relevant Curriculum.* Ford Foundation Publication. New York: Praeger Publishers, 1970.

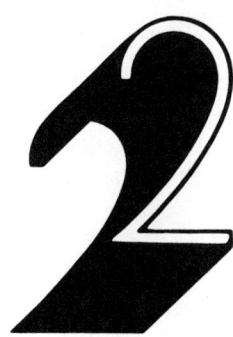

ABOUT VALUES CLARIFICATION

VALUES, VALUES EVERYWHERE . . .

Let's face it, there is no place to hide from your values. Everything you do and say reflects them. Even what you do *not* say and do reflects them.

For example, when you sell something—like a used car—how important is what you choose to tell the potential buyer? Deciding what to say about all the defects in that old heap may not lead to so deep a dilemma for some, but the way you make up your mind about what to say is part of a life-long search for the meaning and significance of living.

Let us telescope in on this situation a little further. You and the potential buyer of your car are just stepping up to the old heap. Some fascinating issues are about to unfold.

Are you about to tell the person at your side everything you possibly can about what is wrong with the car? (We assume you have mentioned all the good points.) Think about that. For each unfavorable point you tell that person, the risk increases that you will eventually sell your car for less money than you'd hoped to reap from the sale—if you sell it at all. Further, if he or she begins to hear an enormous list of things that are wrong with the car, a lightning-quick change of heart may ensue. The purchase may begin to look just too unappealing.

So, where do you draw the line? We always hear the phrase "Honesty is the best policy." Do you think that principle holds true in this situation? Will you decide to tell the interested party anything he or she asks, but hold back information that hasn't been requested? Or, will you decide upon a more complex solution to this personal/moral issue by adopting a double standard? You may want to spill the beans to the person looking at your car if he or she is a good friend or neighbor, but play it cosy with a person who stopped by in response to a newspaper ad.

You might refine your decision even further: What if that person looking at your car is an automobile dealer? You might now consider a third standard. You might feel that if this dealer isn't shrewd enough to spot the defects, then let the buyer truly beware.

Another variation on the theme is also possible as you grapple with this values issue . . . say you know that the brakes need relining right now, and in an emergency, the car would take a dangerously long time to stop. It's even possible, you calculate, that sometime during the next month the linings will wear down so fine that the car might not stop at all.

Of course, on the other side of the fence, the prospective buyer is also engaging in an internal values dialogue. He or she most likely is chewing on a number of these questions: Do I trust the seller? How honest should I be with the seller in terms of the amount of money I'm willing/able to spend? How important are the following factors to me: economical operation, practicality for carrying passengers, peer-group status, safety, power, aesthetic appeal, brand name, company reputation, durability, initial investment, comfort, pollution effects on the environment, amount of gas consumed?

In using this car-sale example, we are trying to drive home the notion that there are a multitude of values issues inherent in every slice of life, from the seemingly innocuous (e.g. What percentage of defects do I want to reveal? Do I want to watch television?) to the "heavy" (e.g. Shall I get involved in some drugs with my friends? What shall I tell my son/daughter about birth control?). Values clarification is one approach that seeks to help us take the steering wheel in our own lives as we sort through this multitude of values issues.

VALUES CLARIFICATION: IN THE BEGINNING . . .

In the beginning, there was Louis E. Raths, who used the term "values clarification" while teaching at New York University during the late 1950s. He springboarded off John Dewey's thinking about the need to move away from isolated moral lessons about particular virtues, and focus rather on helping students to develop skills in formulating and testing judgments and making choices on their own.[1]

Doctoral candidates flocked to Raths' exciting classes of well over a hundred students. He had the gift of touching them personally, and inspiring them to want to set their own lives in order. His relationship with his wife, his family, and his colleagues reflected his deep commitment to living his own radiant values.

In 1966 Raths collaborated with two of his students, Merrill Harmin and Sidney B. Simon, in writing *Values and Teaching* (Columbus, Ohio: Charles E. Merrill Publishing Co.). This book proved to be a strong catalyst in the opening and growth of the values-clarification approach. In the decade following the publication of this book, Simon, Harmin, Howard Kirschenbaum, and Leland Howe have generated a number of other important books: Simon, Howe, and Kirschenbaum, *Values Clarification: A Handbook of Practical Strategies for Teachers and Students;* Harmin, Kirschenbaum, and Simon, *Clarifying Values Through Subject Matter;* and Simon and Kirschenbaum, *Readings in Values Clarification.* In addition, tens of thousands of educators, counselors, parents, and students have participated in workshops or courses designed to help them develop values-clarifying skills. Organizations such as the National Humanistic Education Center (NHEC) have evolved. NHEC has three kinds of services: a mail-order bookstore offering materials in values clarification and humanistic education; national workshops in values clarification and local in-service consulting programs; and assistance in setting up local support groups for people interested in applying humanistic theory, guidelines, and activities in their lives and jobs.

Many school systems across the country have become involved in values clarification through in-service programs, and curriculum innovations.[2] Many community support services (e.g. drug-education programs) have also taken an active interest in values clarification.

As more and more people have become involved in values clarification, there has been an acceleration in the stretching of the field as well. Theoretical developments,[3] new application of values

---

[1] Norma Joyce Hopp. "The Applicability of Value Clarifying Strategies in Health Education at the Sixth Grade Level." (Ph.D. diss., University of Southern California, 1974). John Dewey. *Moral Principles in Education* (Boston: Houghton Mifflin Co., 1909). John Dewey. *Theory of Valuation.* (Chicago: University of Chicago Press, 1939).

[2] An example is documented in Diane Green, Pat Stewart, and Howard Kirschenbaum, "Training a Large Public School System in Values Clarification," in Simon and Kirschenbaum, *Readings in Values Clarification,* pp. 348-57.

[3] See Howard Kirschenbaum, "Beyond Values Clarification" in Simon and Kirschenbaum, *Readings in Values Clarification,* pp. 92-110; Joel Goodman, "Values Clarification: A Review," in John E. Jones and J. William Pfeiffer, *1976 Annual Handbook for Group Facilitators,* pp. 274-279.

clarification to social issues,[4] adaptations to curriculum development and classroom management,[5] creative integrations with subject matter,[6] and a growing body of research[7] have all contributed to the burgeoning field of values clarification. The second decade of values clarification looks as if it will see the continued growth—in depth and in breadth—of the field.[8]

WHAT'S EVERYBODY RUNNING FOR?...
THE NEED FOR VALUES CLARIFICATION

Some people think that values clarification is a fad that will ultimately get an E on its report card (and will thus fade). However, from our perspective, we see values clarification speaking to many crucial needs within our society and educational system. Let us now take a look at a number of responses to the question: "Why do we need values clarification?".

1. Values are important

Raths et al. (1966, p. 27) note that values are "general guides to behavior" that "give direction to life" and "show what we tend to do with our limited time and energy." In a similar vein, Knapp (1972, pp. 26-27) sees a value as "a guiding force that determines the choices people make in living their life." He reinforces the importance of values in noting that "the student ultimately behaves according to how he perceives the world through the screen of his own attitudes and

---

[4]See Eleanor Morrison and Mila Underhill, *Values in Sexuality;* Joel Goodman, Sidney Simon, and Ron Witort, "Tackling Racism by Clarifying Values," *Today's Education* (January 1973) 37-38; Clifford Knapp, "Teaching Environmental Education with a Focus on Values," in Simon and Kirschenbaum, *Readings in Values Clarification,* pp. 161-74.

[5]See Leland Howe and Mary Martha Howe, *Personalizing Education: Values Clarification and Beyond;* Robert Hawley and Isabel Hawley, *Human Values in the Classroom: A Handbook for Teachers;* Sidney Simon, Robert Hawley, and David Britton, *Composition for Personal Growth: Values Clarification Through Writing.*

[6] E.g. see Edward Betof and Howard Kirschenbaum, "Teaching Health Education with a Focus on Values," National Humanistic Education Center, 1973; Jack Osman, "A Rationale for Using Value Clarification in Health Education," *Journal of School Health* (December 1973): pp. 621-23.

[7]As documented in Howard Kirschenbaum's "Current Research in Values Clarification"; see also Bonnie Berger and Vilma Raettig, *The Applicability of Values Clarification to Cardiac Patient Education;* Norma Joyce Hopp, "The Applicability of Value Clarifying Strategies in Health Education at the Sixth Grade Level," and Jack D. Osman, *The Feasibility of Using Selected Value Clarifying Strategies in a Health Education Course for Future Teachers.*

[8]For some visions of this, see Joel Goodman. "Sid Simon on Values," *Nation's Schools* (December 1973) 39-42; Howard Kirschenbaum, Merrill Harmin, Leland Howe, and Sidney B. Simon, "In Defense of Values Clarification."

values." Berman (1968, pp. 155-156) portrays values as "elements of human experience that are invested with great emotional meaning for people . . . the main source of energy in the operation [of society] . . . also the energy that provides the motivational bases for the behavior of individuals in a wide variety of social contexts." It would be quite myopic for schools to ignore such a vital part of their students' lives, and yet, many schools tend to play ostrich when this issue comes into sight. Focusing on values is something that can be "outa sight," but it should not be ostrich-ized.

2. Old approaches haven't worked

Harmin and Simon (1971) list several of the ineffective, and at times, harmful, ways that schools have attempted to deal with values in the past (when they weren't playing "ostrich"): moralizing, inculcating, modeling, rewarding and punishing, nagging, manipulating, and explaining. Wilgoren (1973, p. 5) quotes studies done by Allport, Festinger, McGinnis, and Sykes that reflect the ineffectiveness of these approaches. Berman (1968, p. 172) offers a reason for this ineffectiveness:

These attempts have been met with more or less success—probably less because most persons do not hear unless they are ready to hear. This readiness usually comes about through an active, dynamic process rather than a passive one.

More serious than their ineffectiveness is the damage that these approaches can inflict. Rogers (1969, p. 247) notes that one outcome has been a "fundamental estrangement of modern man from himself." Raths et al. (1966, pp. 5-6) observe that these approaches have produced students who are apathetic, flighty, very uncertain, very inconsistent, drifting, overconforming, overdissenting, and role-playing. Cole (1972) has written a poem that poignantly depicts some of these effects:

Teacher, teacher, tell me true,
Tell me what I ought to do!

Teacher, teacher, where's my book?
Tell me where I ought to look!

Tell me what to feel and how to think,
When to eat and what to drink.

Tell me what is good and what is bad,
When I'm happy and when I'm sad.

Tell me, tell me, what to do,
Tell me, tell me, what is true.

Make me learn and make me know.
Watch me closely as I come and go.

For I am small and I am weak,
Without your permission I cannot speak.

I cannot learn except by your decree,
Please, I beg you, give knowledge to me.

I am stupid and you are bright.
I am wrong and you are right.

I am bad and you are good.
I must do what you say I should.

Oh teacher, teacher, look what you have done!
I don't believe I'm anyone.

Oh teacher, teacher, can't you see!
Look at what you've done to me!

3. The world is changing

There are not many people around who would disagree with this statement. As Toffler in *Future Shock* and others have so ably shown, our world has been invaded by the future. "And accompanying this future shock has been an equally devastating shock to accepted values. The world around us has changed so quickly that the world within us has not had time to catch up. Our values rug is constantly pulled out from under us and we are left confused."[9] Values clarification is one approach that seeks to help us deal with the emerging and often rugged challenges of modern life. It is not *the* way, nor is it a magic wand, (we are slightly suspicious of anyone who would say that he or she has "the answer")—but it can be an extremely helpful tool for us as we soar into the future.

4. Confusion abounds and binds

Given the nature of our changing world and the observation that traditional methods of focusing on values have not worked, many young people and adults today are confused about an array of issues. They often feel as if their hands are tied as they confront questions in such areas as:

friendship	religion	holidays
family	death	future plans
sexuality	politics	drugs
love	race	time
work	ecology	money
leisure	honesty	safety
nutrition	war	sex roles

[9]Sidney B. Simon and Joel B. Goodman, "Values Shock," *Adult Leader* (September, October, November, 1973): 16.

13 ABOUT VALUES CLARIFICATION   Chapter 2

This confusion is compounded when one receives mixed and often conflicting messages from such sources as the home, the church, the peer group, the school, and the media. Students are told in school to brush after every meal, but they rarely see adults following that rule. Students are told that smoking cigarettes can lead to lung cancer, but the media tell them that smoking will get them an attractive mate.

As Charlie Brown of *Peanuts* fame says, "In the book of life, the answers are not in the back." To deal with the values questions and areas, we all need skills in self-literacy: the ability to read "the books" within ourselves and to arrive at our own values decisions. Values clarification is a deliberate approach that seeks to liberate people from the confusion that binds them.

5. Is it always right to be right?

The title of the film of the same name (available from the Espousal Center, 554 Lexington Avenue, Waltham, Mass. 02154) alerts us to another need for values clarification. Just as there can be intrapersonal confusion about values, so can there be interpersonal conflict and confusion. Values can be so highly charged that they can lead a person to stop listening to another who has a different point of view. Worse yet, it may lead one to disrespect, hurt, and/or become polarized from others who are different. This distancing between people manifests itself in a number of ways . . . you're either a hawk or a dove (and never the twain shall meet), you're either *for* busing or *against* busing, you're either a "jock" or a "greaser," you're either over thirty or under thirty, and so on.

It is crucial that our schools equip students with the skills they need in order to live in a pluralistic society. We can ill afford to have student-student and student-teacher polarization. Values clarification is a process that encourages people to *listen* to one another and to respect the humanness in each of us. This does not mean that you will have to agree with everyone else—in fact, conflict can provide a wonderful cutting edge for growth and for consideration of alternatives.

6. Schools have a goals gap

In working with school systems around the country, we have been struck by the incredible difference between what schools would like to do and what they are likely to do. Just take a look at the philosophy or goals of your school or school system. Inevitably, you will find such items as: the school shall help students to develop critical thinking skills, to develop respect for other people and ideas, to enhance their self-concept, to be able to solve "real" problems. These goals all sound very good, and most people would probably reach consensus on them quickly.

Unfortunately, if we look closely, a big difference often exists between the school's rhetoric and its actions—schools rarely are conscious of or conscientious about developing programs and curricula that would speak to these goals. On the other hand, schools are extremely conscious and conscientious about helping students to learn the 3 R's.

Terry Borton wastes no words in talking about this gap:

> There are two sections to almost every school's statement of educational objectives—one for real, one for show. The first, the real one, talks about academic excellence, subject mastery, and getting into college or a job. The other discusses the human purpose of school-values, feelings, personal growth, the full and happy life. It is included because everyone knows that it is important, and that it ought to be central to the life of every school. But it is only for show. Everyone knows how little schools have done about it.[10]

Now, we do not advocate the elimination of traditional subject matter from the schools—we think it is crucial for students to have the basic reading, 'riting, and 'rithmetic skills in order to get along in this world. But we also think it is crucial for them to have the basic human skills.[11] They are not mutually exclusive—in fact, they could be complementary!

Above all, the most important question with regard to goals is, "Whom is the school serving?" The matter often boils down, as one teacher put it, to a matter of teaching students or teaching subject matter. It's unfortunate that many teachers are under pressure "to get to 1860 by the end of the semester," and in the process often lose students' attention by the middle of the semester. Witness the teacher who came across this remark on a student's paper: "Sometimes I wish I was dead." If the teacher had responded only to the grammar on this paper (e.g. correcting "was" to "were"), then he might have easily "lost" this student both figuratively and literally.

7. We're in a race against runaway devaluation

On your mark, get set . . . We are not talking here about monetary devaluation, but the devaluation of people. We have been appalled to find that many students cannot identify a single success they have had or a positive quality about themselves. We have been equally dismayed to work with groups of students who could identify in a five-minute period more than two hundred killer phrases that are a regular part of their vocabulary; killer phrases, or put-downs, include such remarks as "That's dumb!," "You're weird!," "That's a stupid idea—we tried it

---

[10]Terry Borton, "Reach, Touch, and Teach," *Saturday Review,* 18 January 1969, pp. 56–58, 69–70.

[11]Howard Kirschenbaum calls them "life skills" in "What Is Humanistic Education," *Humanistic Education Quarterly* (May 1973): 3–4.

last year!" These killer phrases are so ingrained in our patterns of interaction that we even begin saying them to ourselves—about ourselves; hence, the inability of students to focus on their "good" traits.

The *Peanuts* gang offers another illustration of devaluation:

One day, Linus notes that Charlie Brown has been a really dedicated baseball manager, always giving 110% to the team. Linus suggests that the team show their appreciation to Charlie by giving him a testimonial dinner. Lucy responds by doubting that he deserves a whole testimonial dinner, and recommends instead that they give him a testimonial snack.[12]

We have seen too many people who are starving for even a testimonial nibble. Essentially, the race against devaluation is an effort to erase self-concept malnutrition. Values clarification is one process that attempts to have people nourish themselves by focusing on their values and on their value.

8. Values clarification is a holistic, skills-oriented approach

Unlike other approaches to working with values, values clarification addresses its useful theory and activities to the whole person. Kirschenbaum (1973, p. 10) elaborates:

It is interesting that, while some existentialists and others say that our actions reveal our values, there are others who equate our beliefs and opinions with our values. Still others see values as synonymous with attitudes and preferences. Values clarification is unique in that it sees the valuing process as involving feelings, thoughts, and actions, not one to the exclusion of the others.

Another distinguishing characteristic is that values clarification emphasizes the *process* of *valuing,* rather than the content of values. Its focus is reflected in the quotation, "If you give me a fish, I'll eat tonight. If you teach me *how to* fish, I'll eat for a lifetime." As a preventive, positive approach to mental and emotional health (dealing with the whole person), values clarification helps people to develop skills (how to's) in four areas: the cognitive (thinking), the affective (feeling), the active (behaving), and the interpersonal (communicating).

Cognitive skills

1 Choosing freely (e.g. dealing with peer pressure).
2 Choosing from among alternatives.
3 Choosing with an awareness of the consequences of one's choices.
4 Being aware of patterns in one's life.
5 Thinking critically (analyzing, synthesizing, drawing inferences).
6 Ideating (the ability to generate ideas and alternatives).

---

[12] Joel B. Goodman and Marie Hartwell Walker, "Values Clarification: Helping People to Feel More Value-Able," *Ohio's Health,* 28, no. 9 (September 1975): 11-15.

Affective skills

7 Identifying and acknowledging feelings as one data source in making decisions.
8 Legitimizing one's intuition as another possible data source in making decisions.
9 Focusing on what one prizes and cherishes.

Active skills

10 Acting on one's choices (moving from insight to behavioral change).
11 Goal-setting.
12 Culling out the inconsistencies between what one would like to do and what one is likely to do.

Interpersonal skills

13 Publicly affirming one's choices where appropriate; sending "I" messages.
14 Empathic listening.
15 Resolving conflict situations.
16 Asking clarifying questions.
17 Community-building (building on commonalities; respecting differences).
18 Validating (focusing on the "positive" in self and others; avoiding killer phrases).

VALUES CLARIFICATION: A NUTSHELL SUMMARY

If asked to give a 25-words-or-more definition of values clarification, here is what it might look like: Values clarification = one approach to improving the quality of life that involves people developing cognitive, affective, active, and interpersonal skills: seeks to help people: (1) clarify their values; (2) feel more valuable; and (3) appreciate the lovability and capability of self and others.

REFERENCES

Berman, Louise. *New Priorities in the Classroom.* Columbus, Ohio: Charles E. Merrill Publishing Co., 1968.

Cole, Henry. "Tell Me, Teacher." Handout at Creative Problem Solving Institute, Creative Education Foundation, Buffalo, N.Y., 1972.

Harmin, Merrill, and Simon, Sidney B. "Values." *Teacher's Handbook.* Edited by Dwight Allen and Eli Seifman. Glenview, Illinois: Scott, Foresman, 1971, pp. 690-98.

_____; Kirschenbaum, Howard; and Simon, Sidney B. *Clarifying Values Through Subject Matter.* Minneapolis, Minnesota: Winston Press, Inc., 1973.

Hawley, Robert C.; Simon, Sidney B.; and Britton, David D. *Composition for Personal Growth: Values Clarification Through Writing.* New York: Hart Publishing Co., 1973.

_____; and Hawley, Isabel. *Human Values in the Classroom.* New York: Hart Publishing Co. Inc., 1976.

Howe, Leland, and Howe, Mary Martha. *Personalizing Education: Values Clarification and Beyond.* New York: Hart Publishing Co., 1975.

Kirschenbaum, Howard. "Beyond Values Clarification." *Humanistic Education Quarterly* (October 1973): 1-14.

_____. "Current Research in Values Clarification." Saratoga Springs, N.Y.: National Humanistic Education Center, 1975.

_____; Harmin, Merrill; Howe, Leland; and Simon, Sidney B. "In Defense of Values Clarification." Saratoga Springs, N.Y.: National Humanistic Education Center, 1975.

Knapp, Clifford. "Attitudes and Values in Environmental Education." *Journal of Environmental Education* (Summer 1972): 26-29.

Morrison, Eleanor, and Underhill, Mila. *Values in Sexuality.* New York: Hart Publishing Co., 1974.

Pfeiffer, J. William, and Jones, John E. *1976 Annual Handbook for Group Facilitators.* Iowa City, Iowa: University Associates, 1976.

Raths, Louis E.; Harmin, Merrill; and Simon, Sidney B. *Values and Teaching.* Columbus, Ohio: Charles E. Merrill Publishing Co., 1966.

Rogers, Carl. *Freedom to Learn.* Columbus, Ohio: Charles E. Merrill Publishing Co., 1969.

Simon, Sidney B.; Howe, Leland; and Kirschenbaum, Howard. *Values Clarification: A Handbook of Practical Strategies for Teachers and Students.* New York: Hart Publishing Co., 1972.

_____; and Kirschenbaum, Howard. *Readings in Values Clarification.* Minneapolis, Minnesota: Winston Press, 1973.

Toffler, Alvin. *Future Shock.* New York: Random House, Inc., 1970.

Wilgoren, Richard. "The Relationship Between the Self-Concept of Pre-Service Teachers and Two Methods of Teaching Value Clarification." Doctoral dissertation, University of Massachusetts, 1973.

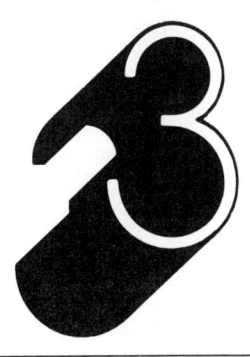

1+1=3: VALUES CLARIFICATION + HEALTH EDUCATION

THE DYNAMIC DUO

Values clarification and health education have been developing an increasingly stronger and synergetic alliance in the quest for a better quality of life. Values clarification is a natural *process* that can be used to focus on many of the values-rich *content* areas in health education. Many young people (and adults) are tackling healthy questions that are ripe for values exploration:

Sexuality. How can I improve my relationship with my spouse? What and how can I teach my children about sexual feelings? In what ways can I better give and receive affection, caring, and love? Where do I stand with regard to sex roles—now and in the future?

Drugs. To what extent do I want to rely on drugs (aspirin, cigarettes, alcohol, pot, and so on) in my life? What can I do to deal with the peer-group pressure I encounter around drugs? What are some alternative ways of getting "high" in my life? Are drugs really a cop-out or a legitimate pleasure trip?

Family, family life. I wonder what will become of my family when I leave home? How can I get my parents to respect my point of

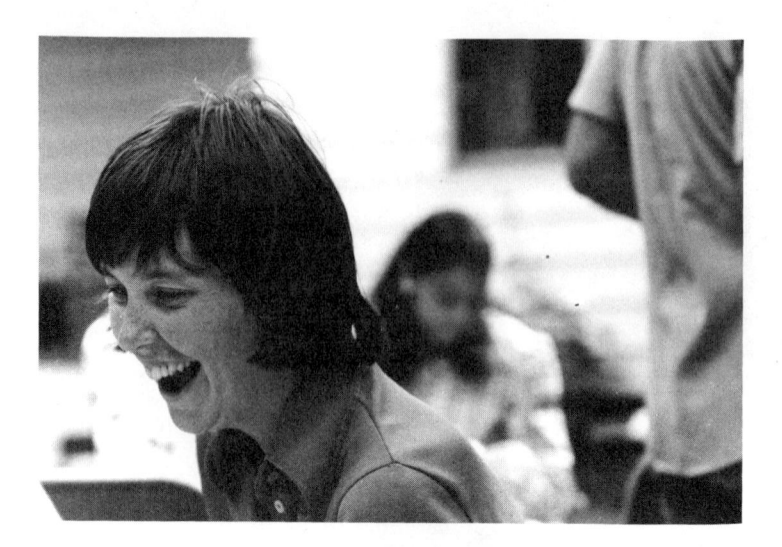

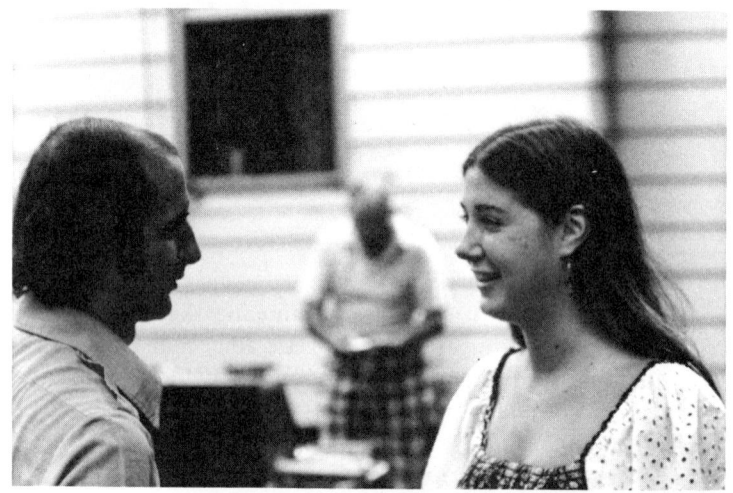

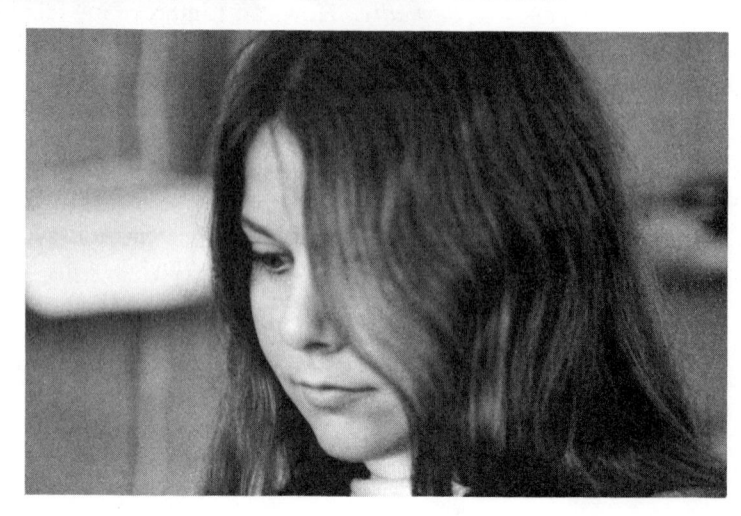

view? How can I get my children to respect my point of view? What can I do to get along better with my brother and sister?

Nutrition. Where do I fit in and what responsibility do I have with regard to the world food crisis? How can I cut down on sweets between meals? Do I want to consider becoming a vegetarian? What might I do if a loved one were not eating well?

Safety. Is it worth my time to put on seat belts when I'm in a car? What kinds of dares would I be willing to take? What kinds of dares would I refuse to take? How could I make my home environment safer for my young children?

Death, dying, and growing old. What am I now doing to help myself live a long, healthy life? Do I believe in "mercy killing"? Do I want to have a funeral, be cremated, donate my body to science, or what? If I had one year to live, what would I do with it?

Environment, ecology. Shall I buy a used car that pollutes, or a more-expensive, new car with pollution controls? What can I do at home to conserve electricity/energy? What might I do if I saw someone littering? What might I do to improve the environment in my community?

VALUES CLARIFICATION: MOVING FROM HEALTH INFORMATION TO HEALTH EDUCATION

These kinds of questions, which people face every day, are not ones that "have an answer in the back of the book." A growing number of individuals are recognizing that the factual approach and the scare-tactic approach to health are at best ineffective, and at worst, counterproductive.[1] David Page's quotation summarizes the dilemma: "If to possess knowledge alone is to be educated, then an encyclopedia is better educated than a person."

Louis Raths posed a series of questions that creates a bridge between health information and health education. He would start by asking "What is the function of information?" The rhetorical answer would always be, "Well, the function of information is to inform." He followed this with the query, "To inform what?" The answer he cherished was: to inform your values, so that what you studied as content would show up in your life.

[1] See Bernard Bard, "The Failure of Our School Drug Abuse Programs," *Phi Delta Kappan* (December 1975): 251-55; Nancy Faber, "Facts Alone Are Not Enough," *Learning* (February 1973): 10-14; Lenny Glynn, "Doing the Job on Drugs," *Media and Methods* (March 1973): 40-42, 56, 58.

Recent years have seen a growing movement toward a values-clarification approach to health education. Witness the following publications:

Howard Kirschenbaum's "Clarifying Values at the Family Table," in Simon and Kirschenbaum's *Readings in Values Clarification,* pp. 265-70.

Jack D. Osman's "The Feasibility of Using Selected Value Clarifying Strategies in a Health Education Course for Future Teachers." Unpublished doctoral dissertation, Ohio State University, 1971.

Sidney B. Simon's "Dinner Table Learning," *Colloquy* (December 1971): 34-37.

Joel Goodman and Laurie Hawkins's "Value Clarification: Meeting a Challenge in Education," *Colloquy* (May 1972),: 18-22.

Paul Kelley and Gladys Conroy's "A Promotive Health Plan Preventing Alcohol and Drug Abuse in the Schools," *Arizona Medicine* (January 1972).

Clifford E. Knapp's "Attitudes and Values in Environmental Education," *Journal of Environmental Education* (Summer 1972): 26-29.

Clifford E. Knapp's "The Environment: Children Explore Their Values," *Instructor Magazine* (March 1972): 116-18.

Clifford E. Knapp's "Teaching Environmental Education with a Focus on Values," in Simon and Kirschenbaum's *Readings in Values Clarification,* pp. 161-74.

Floyd D. Rees's "Teaching the Valuing Process in Sex Education," *School Health Review* (March-April 1972): 2-4.

Sidney B. Simon's "Election Year and Dinner Table Learning," *Colloquy* (October 1972): 23-25.

Merrill Harmin, Howard Kirschenbaum, and Sidney B. Simon's *Clarifying Values Through Subject Matter* (Minneapolis: Winston Press, 1973), pp. 85-88. (See especially the chapter on "Family Life and Sex Education").

Jack D. Osman's "A Rationale for Using Value Clarification in Health Education," *Journal of School Health* (December 1973) pp. 621-23.

Jack D. Osman's "Teaching Nutrition with a Focus on Values," *Nutrition News* (April 1973).

School Health Review, January-February 1974 (Special issue devoted to articles on values clarification).

Norma Joyce Hopp's "The Applicability of Value Clarifying Strategies in Health Education at the Sixth Grade Level." Unpublished doctoral dissertation, University of Southern California, 1974.

Bonnie Berger and Vilma Raettig's "The Applicability of Values Clarification to Cardiac Patient Education." Unpublished master's thesis, Loma Linda University, 1974.

Jack D. Osman's "Value Growth Through Drug Education," *School Health Review* (January-February 1974): 25-30.

Norma Joyce Hopp's "V.C.and the Sixth Grade," *School Health Review* (January-February 1974): 34-35.

Joel Goodman and Marie Hartwell Walker's "Values Clarification: Helping People to Feel More Value-Able," *Ohio's Health* (September 1975): 11-15.

Floyd D. Rees's "Teaching Values Through Health Education," *School Health Review* (February 1970): 15-17.

Sidney B. Simon's "Promoting the Search for Values," *School Health Review* (February 1971): 21-24.

Cynthia Parris's "Operation Outreach: A New Dimension in Drug Abuse Education." Paper presented at American Public Health Association Convention, San Francisco, November 1973.

Eleanor Morrison and Mila Underhill's *Values in Sexuality* (New York: Hart Publishing Co., 1974.

Jerrold S. Greenberg's "Behavior Modification and Values Clarification and Their Research Implications," *The Journal of School Health* (February 1975): 91-95.

Joyce W. Hopp's "Values Clarification and the School Nurse," *The Journal of School Health* (September 1975) 410-413.

Donald A. Read and Howard E. Munson's "Resolution of One's Sexual Self: An Important First Step for Sexuality Educators," *The Journal of School Health* (January 1976) 31-34.

William Blokker, et al.,"Values Clarification and Drug Abuse," *Health Education* (March-April 1976) 6-8.

Donald A. Read and Howard E. Munson, *Sexuality Education: A Reassessment of Values Through The Humanistic Process.* To be published by Prentice-Hall, Inc.

Sidney B. Simon and Joel B. Goodman's "A Study of Death Through the Celebration of Life" *Learning* (March 1976): 70-74.

Joel B. Goodman, et al.,"Toward A Quality of Living," New York: *JC Penney Consumer Education Modules,* 1976.

VALUES CLARIFICATION AND HEALTH EDUCATION: WHERE AND HOW

One of the major strengths of values clarification is that it is an incredibly flexible and highly adaptable approach. It has been and can be used in a wide variety of arenas: (1) providing the individual student with opportunities to do some private reflection; (2) the teacher and student engaging in a one-on-one values exploration; (3) students working in small groups on clarifying values; (4) the entire class working on values issues and skills; (5) a faculty taking time to clarify personal and/or professional values; (6) a counselor or school nurse supporting a student in the valuing process; (7) a family working on some values issues of interest/concern; (8) teaching students to be peer and/or cross-age counselors (using the valuing skills in student-support groups or "family" groups); (9) cross-age, cross-role groups (e.g. students, parents, teachers, administrators) meeting to promote communication skills and to develop respect for others and their values; (10) courses for students in values-rich areas (e.g. "Family Living," "Making a Life, Making a Living: Future Plans and Career Education," "Friendship," "Environmental Education")—these often appear as electives;[2] (11) student-generated interest groups; (12) individual student projects; (13) in nurse-patient relationships.

Given the contexts just mentioned, there are a number of modes (how to's) for integrating values clarification into health education. These include: (1) use of clarifying responses; (2) use of values-clarification activities; and/or (3) three-level teaching and learning. It is crucial to recognize that these modes can be interdependent and complementary.

Clarifying responses

This is one of the basic tools in the values-clarification repertoire.[3] As with the other modes, the basic aim of the clarifying response is to help the individual(s) (e.g. student, family member, patient, and so on) to examine his or her own life and values. The beauty of the clarifying response is that it can be used spontaneously (on the spur of the moment, in response to a student's statement) and/or as part of the processing of a structured activity. In fact, the clarifying response is *more* important than the activity itself.[4]

Clarifying responses often meet the following kinds of criteria: (1) They plant seeds: they are often brief comments that encourage the individual to reflect on his/her thoughts, feelings, and/or behaviors. Many times they stand alone, although they can lead to further discussion; (2) They do not have a "right answer" behind them. Effective and ethical clarifying responses avoid moralizing. Responses that begin with the words "Don't you think that . . . " are often read as moralistic, and the student will spend more time trying to psyche you out than in clarifying for himself/herself; (3) They aim to help people develop the cognitive, affective, active, and interpersonal skills listed in the previous chapter; they seek to help individuals "learn how to fish" (valuing) rather than "give them a fish" (impose values).

[2]Sidney B. Simon and Joel Goodman; "Values Clarification and the School Psychologist."
[3]Louis E. Raths, Merrill Harmin, and Sidney B. Simon; *Values and Teaching,* Columbus, Ohio: Charles E. Merrill Publishing Co., 1966, pp. 51-82.
[4]Joel B. Goodman and Marie Hartwell Walker, "Affective Ed—A Means, Not an End," *Learning,* 4, no. 5 (January 1976): 52.

Raths, Harmin, and Simon (1966, pp. 55-65) offer examples of a number of clarifying responses that meet the above criteria:

1. Where do you suppose you first got that idea?
2. How long have you felt that way?
3. Are you getting help from anyone? Do you need more help? Can I help?
4. Are you the only one in your crowd who feels this way?
5. Is there any rebellion in your choice?
6. What else did you consider before you picked this?
7. How long did you look around before you decided?
8. Was it a hard decision? What went into the final decision?
9. Are there some reasons behind your choice?
10. What choices did you reject before you settled on your present idea or action?
11. What's really good about this choice that makes it stand out from the other possibilities?
12. What would be the consequences of each alternative available?
13. Have you thought about this very much? How did your thinking go?
14. Is this what I understand you to say . . . [interpret the statement]?
15. What assumptions are involved in your choice?
16. Is what you say consistent with what you said earlier?
17. Where will it lead?
18. For whom are you doing this?
19. What will you have to do? What are your first steps?
20. To whom else did you talk?
21. Have you weighed your choice fully?
22. Are you glad you feel that way?
23. Why is it important to you? What purpose does it serve?
24. Is it something you really prize?
25. In what way would life be different without it?
26. Would you be willing to sign a petition supporting that idea?
27. Are you saying that you believe . . . [repeat the idea]?
28. Do people know that you believe that way?
29. Are you willing to stand up and be counted for that?
30. I hear what you are for . . . now, is there anything you can do about it?
31. Are you willing to put some of your time, energy, and resources behind that idea?
32. Have you made any plans to do more than you have already done?
33. Who has influenced you on this?
34. Where will this lead you? How far are you willing to go?
35. How has it already affected your life? How will it affect you in the future?
36. How long do you think you will continue?
37. How did you decide which had priority?
38. Did you run into any difficulty?
39. Will you do it again?
40. Are there some other things you can do that are like it?

A well-timed and appropriate clarifying response can often help a person to make progress in tackling alive/life/living issues (e.g. sexuality, drugs, safety, nutrition, family, death and dying, ecology). The focus for you is on raising the "right question" rather than on providing the "right answer."

Here are several clarifying questions for you, the reader: In the situations or vignettes listed below, what kinds of clarifying responses would you like to use? What kinds of clarifying responses would you be likely to use? What are the consequences of each of these possible clarifying responses? How would you feel if you were on the receiving end of these clarifying responses? When do you think that clarifying responses are not appropriate (e.g. when sending an "I" message might be better)?

a In a health-education class, one of the students declares that he does not ever want to get married.
b When riding in the car, you notice that one of your children always wears her seat belt and your other child never does.
c During lunch break, you see several students littering on the school grounds.
d In a discussion on nutrition, several students express a desire to become vegetarians.
e A student approaches you in the hall and asks you to sign a petition in favor of setting up a student smoking lounge.
f A student approaches you in the hall and asks you to sign a petition in favor of abolishing smoking in the school (by both teachers and students).

Values-clarification activities

Values clarification has become so widespread in large measure because of its exciting, involving, meaningful, and enjoyable activities. Of the hundreds of activities that have been developed, some are what we call "bread-and-butter" strategies (they can be used over time, adapted and stretched in many ways) while others are "one-time" strategies (their major impact is in a single use).

Values-clarification activities can be employed either congruently or confluently. By this, we mean that the teacher can incorporate them in a thematic approach (e.g. a values unit or course on "drugs," "human sexuality," or "ecology," where the emphasis is on students examining their values and developing valuing skills—the congruent use), and/or integrate them with "traditional" subject matter (the confluent use—e.g. in studying medical advances in a science class, the teacher could springboard off the subject-matter content and introduce a values-clarification activity that would encourage students to clarify their values about death, dying, nutrition, and the positive/negative consequences of drugs).

It is *crucial* for us to remember not to equate values clarification with its activities. As mentioned earlier, the activities are only one vehicle. In fact, if we looked closely, we would see that the activities are simply extensions and elaborations of effective clarifying responses.

In chapter 4 we offer specific examples of five bread-and-butter strategies that could be used to focus on any values-rich area: values-voting questions, rank-ordering, continua, inventories, and moral dilemmas.

Three-level teaching and learning

The reality of most schools today is that there is a great deal of pressure (on teachers and on students) to focus on "subject matter." What, then, is the teacher to do who says, "Yes, I believe in the theory, guidelines, and practical activities involved in values clarification, but where, oh, where do I 'fit them in' "?

One way is to look at learning as a tripartite wheel which includes the following elements:

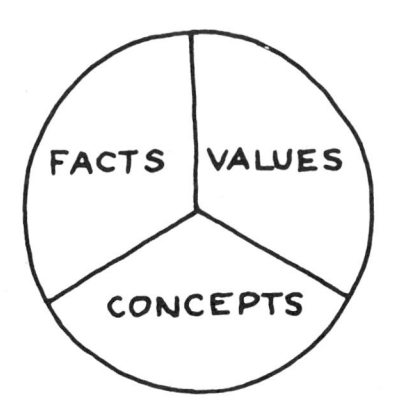

FACTS / VALUES / CONCEPTS

Almost any subject matter can be taught on all three levels. For example, the following excerpt might appear in a science text:

The human being is made up of oxygen, nitrogen, phosphorous, hydrogen, carbon, and calcium. There are also 12½ gallons of water, enough iron to make a small nail, about a salt shaker full of salt, and enough sugar to make one small cube. If one were to put all of this together and try to sell it, the thing would be worth about one dollar.

A teacher might ask the following factual-level questions:

1 How much water is there in the human body?
2 True or false: The body contains enough sugar to make two small cubes.
3 How much money could you receive if you tried to sell the "contents" of your body?

28 HEALTH EDUCATION: THE SEARCH FOR VALUES

A teacher might also ask the following conceptual-level questions:

1 What is the difference between a liquid, a gas, and a solid?
2 What is the relationship between density and volume?
3 How is water formed?

A teacher who is interested in helping students to develop valuing skills might go beyond the questions just enumerated and have students consider the following:

1 Do you believe you are worth more than one dollar? Explain.
2 If you were the late J. Paul Getty, would you be willing to pay a $3.4 million ransom for your grandson?
3 When do you feel most worthwhile? With whom do you feel most worthwhile?
4 Can you think of some ways to help others feel that they are worth more?
5 Some students feel that they are not worth even a dollar. What might you say to people who feel like this?

The values-level questions have two distinguishing characteristics. First, each of them contains the word "you." The questions ask students, "What has this information got to do with you, your life, your values?" In this sense, they are genuine clarifying responses. Second, each question avoids moralizing. There are no "right answers" to values-level questions. What is important here is to help students become self-literate: to find their own "answers" in the "book" within themselves.

One of the strengths of values clarification is its adaptability. Almost any subject matter or values-rich area can be explored on all three levels. All the students need is a stimulus (which can be a picture, a song, a filmstrip, an article from a newspaper, or an excerpt from a textbook), followed by the appropriate questions. In fact, this is the formula for one of the values clarification activities in the appendix, the values sheet.

values sheet = provocative stimulus + clarifying questions

Drawing from Harmin, Kirschenbaum, and Simon's *Clarifying Values Through Subject Matter* (pp. 106–07), we now present you, the reader, with the following values sheet:

What is worth teaching? Much of what is taught in schools is so remote from students' lives that it would be a travesty to try to teach that material on the values level. Sugar-coating an irrelevant curriculum with values questions is not the way to clarify and develop values. It will fool no one for very long. Therefore, before teachers begin to find ways to teach their subject area of the values level, they must ask themselves some serious questions. . . . There is no foolproof way of determining what to include in a curriculum or what to eliminate from it. Each teacher must reach this decision on his own, and very likely this will be an ongoing decision. Many teachers will continue to teach subject matter which they regard as valuable, even if it has no apparent relation to how students live their lives. To teach with a focus on values does not mean to eliminate these areas from the curriculum. It is a question of balance. Each teacher must decide which areas of his subject he will teach in order to focus on values and which areas of his subject he will teach for other purposes.

1   Why are you teaching this subject area?
2   Do you really believe your students need to have this knowledge or these skills?
3   If you had no restraints or mandates imposed on you, what would you freely choose to teach?
4   How does each area you are considering teaching relate to your students' lives?
5   What are the real values dilemmas present in the subjects and themes you teach?

We think it is of vital importance for people using values clarification to ask themselves (continuously) these kinds of questions. Meanwhile, here are some additional examples of three-level teaching/learning to whet your appetite while you continue to munch on the food for thought just offered:

Drugs

Ten years ago today, the Surgeon General of the United States issued a report citing cigarette smoking as a major hazard to life and health. Yet the anniversary of that historic 387-page document finds cigarette sales at an all-time high, per capita consumption increasing and 3000 teenagers becoming new smokers each day . . . about 40% of men and 30% of women are current cigarette smokers . . . The tobacco industry, while continuing to maintain that cigarettes are not the health hazards they are made out to be, has nonetheless catered to the public demand for less tar and nicotine.[5]

Factual questions:

1   How many teenagers become new smokers every day?
2   True or false: More men smoke than women.
3   What is it about cigarettes that makes them harmful?

[5]*Springfield Union,* 11 January, 1974.

Conceptual questions:

1. What does "per capita" mean?
2. What is a "habit?" What are some habits that people have other than cigarette smoking?
3. Why has cigarette smoking increased since the Surgeon General's report?

Values questions:

1. Do you plan to smoke when you are a teenager? What attracts you to smoking? What would discourage you from smoking?
2. Do you think society ought to make cigarettes illegal?
3. Do you have any ideas on how to protect the rights of both smokers and nonsmokers?
4. What recommendations would you have for someone who wanted to quit smoking but didn't know how to do it? Have you ever given up a habit that you enjoyed but that was not good for you? How did you do it?
5. If you just found out that you had one year to live, how would you spend your time?[6]

Ecology, environment

In Malaysia recently, in an effort to kill off mosquitoes, American technologists sprayed woods and swamplands with DDT. Result? Cockroaches, which ate poisoned mosquitoes, were so slowed in their reactions that they could be eaten by a variety of tree-climbing lizard which, sickened in turn, could be eaten by cats, which promptly died of insecticide poisoning. The cats having died, the rat population began to increase; as rats multiplied, so did fleas: hence the rapid spread of bubonic plague in Malaysia. But this is not all. The tree-climbing lizards, having died, could no longer eat an insect which consumed the straw thatching of the natives' huts. So as Malaysians died of plague, their roofs literally caved in above their heads.[7]

Factual questions:

1. Fill in the blank: _____ ate the poisoned mosquitoes.
2. On what continent did the events described above occur?
3. Check the true statements: The Malaysians' roofs caved in because of heavy rainfall. Americans sprayed DDT in the woods and swamplands of Malaysia. Bubonic plague spread in Malaysia.

[6]Excerpted from Joel B. Goodman and Marie Hartwell Walker, "Values Clarification: Helping People to Feel More Value-Able," *Ohio's Health.* 28, no. 9 (September 1975): 11-15.

[7]Peter A. Gunter, North Texas State University, in *The Living Wilderness,* Spring, 1970.

Learning Through Doing . . .

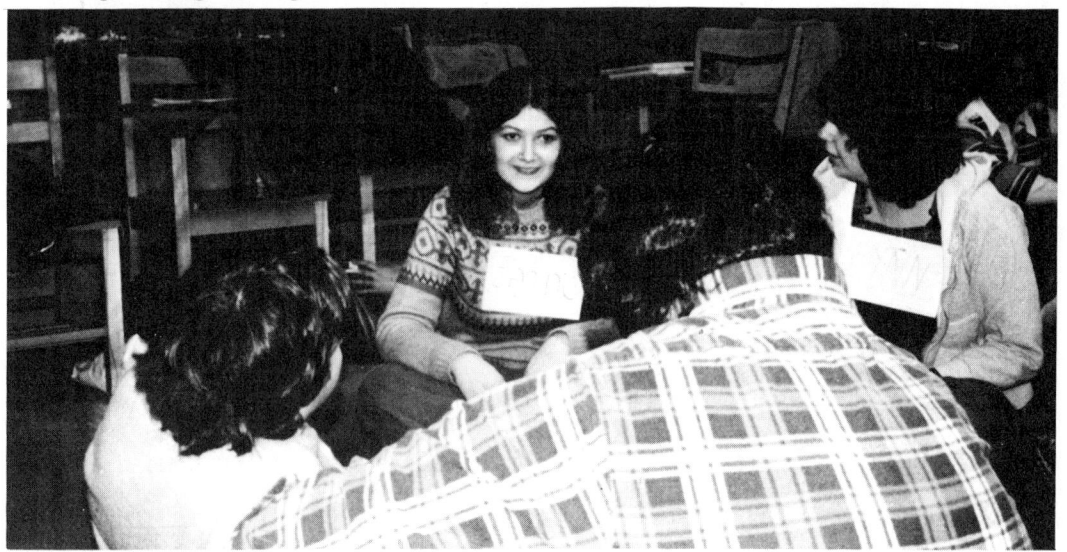

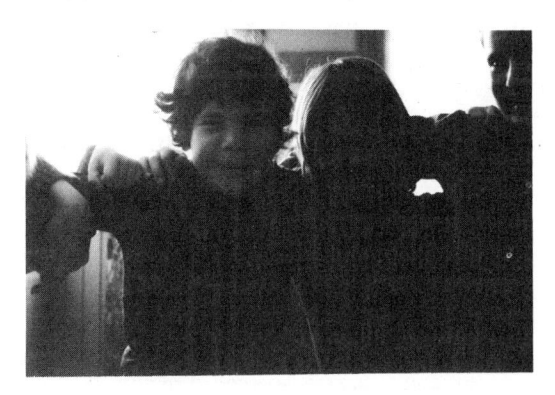

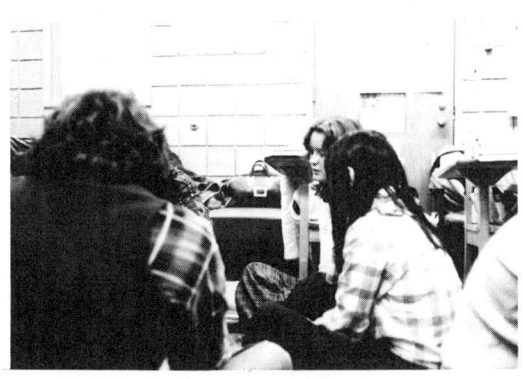

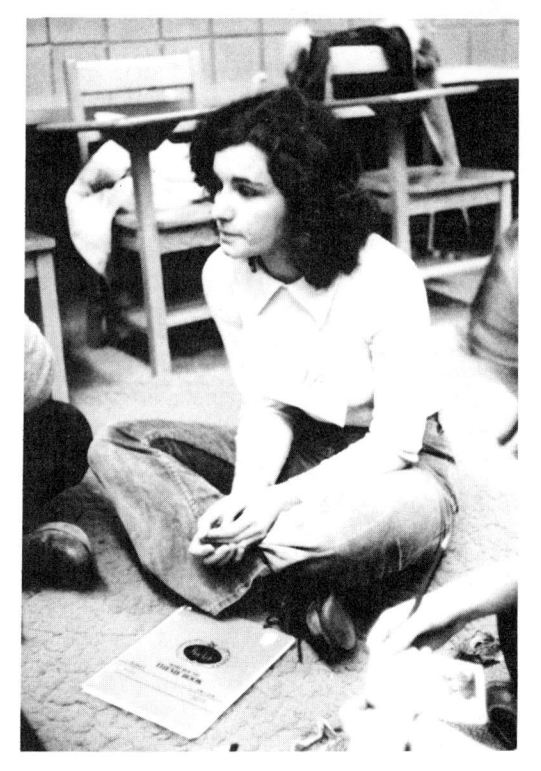

Conceptual questions:

1. Discuss the concept of "food chain." Give examples.
2. What are some of the ways of describing the relationship between humans and nature, between human technology and environment?
3. Compare the life cycle of the cat with the life cycle of its prey, the rat.

Values questions:

1. Write your reaction to the paragraph preceding on ecology and environment. Do it quickly. Don't even write full sentences.
2. What implications does this paragraph have for your own life?
3. Can you list some things you did in the past that might well have broken the delicate balance of nature?
4. What changes have you made in your life because of increased awareness of ecological factors?

Death

The family's greatest reluctance over having the treatment at all was the fear that the patient would discover her diagnosis. They had decided in the past that she should never know, and that they would lie to her about her condition so as not to take away her hope and to keep her happy. However, in the last few months her psychological condition had worsened greatly and she was filled with anxiety and worry.[8]

Factual questions:

1. What kind of training does one need to become a doctor?
2. True or false: When one enters a hospital, he or she gives up his/her civil rights.
3. What was the decision in the recent court case on whether to remove or maintain life-supporting measures for Karen Quinlan, a young women who had been lying in a coma for months?

Conceptual questions:

1. What is the relationship between one's physical condition and one's psychological condition?
2. Compare and contrast the rights of a patient in a hospital with the rights of a prisoner in a jail.
3. Discuss the difference between the medical and the religious definitions of "death."

[8]Jerry Avorn. *"Beyond Dying." Harper's,* March 1973, p. 59.

Values questions:

1. Do you feel that there is not enough secrecy, too much secrecy, or just about the right amount of secrecy about death in our society?
2. When a doctor does not inform a patient that he or she is going to die, and the patient's family goes along with this, wo do you think benefits the most—the patient, the family, or the doctor?
3. If someone very close to you—a friend or relative—were hopelessly sick and everyone except this person knew he was going to die, would you or would you not tell him?
4. If your doctor and your family knew that you were going to die, would you prefer that they try to keep up a hopeful attitude, or tell you the truth?
5. If you were going to die, would you volunteer for a therapeutic LSD session if your doctor felt it might help you to better accept your impending death?[9]

A SUMMARY

In this chapter, we have described some of the tools and approaches in the values-clarification repertoire that can help us to move from a health-information program to a health-education program. This movement is an evolutionary one, because as Alvin Eurich notes:

We cannot tolerate another generation that knows so much about preserving and destroying life, but so little about enhancing it. We cannot permit our children to come into their maturity as masters of the atom and of the gene, but ignorant about the ways of the human mind and heart.[10]

REFERENCES

Borton, Terry, *Reach, Touch, and Teach,* New York: McGraw-Hill, Book Co., 1970.

Harmin, Merrill; Kirschenbaum, Howard; and Simon, Sidney B. *Clarifying Values Through Subject Matter,* Minnesota: Winston Press, 1973.

Hawley, Robert, *Human Values in the Classroom,* Amherst, Mass.: Education Research Associates, 1973.

_____, *Value Exploration,* Amherst, Mass.: Education Research Associates, 1974.

_____, and Hawley, Isabel. *A Handbook of Personal Growth Activities for Classroom Use,* Amherst, Mass.: Education Research Associates, 1972.

[9]From a values sheet by Janice Stone.

[10]Quoted in Danforth Foundarion, I.D.E.A. and N.A.S.S.P.'s *An Occasional Paper: Toward a More Relevant Curriculum,* 1970, p. 1.

_____; Simon, Sidney B.; and Britton, David D. *Composition for Personal Growth,* New York: Hart Publishing Co., Inc., 1973.

Raths, Louis; Harmin, Merrill; and Simon, Sidney B. *Values and Teaching,* Columbus, Ohio: Charles E. Merrill Publishing Co., 1966.

Rucker, Roy; Arnspiger, Claude; and Brodbeck, Arthur, *Human Values in Education,* Dubuque, Iowa: Kendall/Hunt Publishing Co., 1969.

Schrank, Jeffrey, *Media in Value Education: A Critical Guide,* Chicago, Ill.: Argus Communications, 1970.

Simon, Sidney B.; Howe, Leland; and Kirschenbaum, Howard. *Values Clarification,* New York: Hart Publishing Co., Inc., 1972.

_____, and Goodman, Joel. "Values Clarification and the School Psychologist," *International Encyclopedia of Neurology, Psychiatry, Psychoanalysis, and Psychology.* In press.

VALUES CLARIFICATION ACTIVITIES: A TASTE FOR SOME BREAD-AND-BUTTER STRATEGIES

As mentioned in chapter 3, one mode for helping students to explore their values in the classroom is through structured experiences. The present chapter includes examples of five values-clarification activities (structured experiences) that can be used to help students explore health-related issues. These activities were chosen because: (1) they are highly adaptable—teachers and students alike can generate, modify, and/or stretch these activities very easily; (2) they reflect some of the basic structures underlying values-clarification activities (hence, the description "bread-and-butter"); (3) they suggest the variety of possible ways to help students develop valuing skills.

The chapter is divided into three sections: (1) values clarification with a focus on human sexuality and family life; (2) values clarification with a focus on drugs; and (3) values clarification with a focus on nutrition. Within each section, we offer examples of applications of each of the following bread and butter strategies: (a) rank-ordering; (b) values-voting; (c) spread of opinion; (d) moral dilemmas; (e) inventory.

We also provide you, the reader, with some space in which to generate your own activities and/or to modify the ones we have presented. We see this chapter solely as a springboard—the examples we suggest are by no means exhaustive—and, in some cases, they may not be appropriate! The most important idea that we can communicate is this: IT IS CRUCIAL THAT YOU BE SENSITIVE TO THE READINESS OF YOUR STUDENTS FOR ANY PARTICULAR ACTIVITY OR CONTENT AREA.

THE PURPOSE OF THE ACTIVITIES

Although students often find these activities to be fun, they are not "for fun." We have a specific objective(s) in mind each and every time we employ a values-clarification activity. In fact, we see these activities speaking directly to the valuing skills mentioned in the previous chapter (the cognitive, the affective, the active, and the interpersonal). Some teachers find it helpful to state the objective of the activity explicitly to the students (beforehand and/or after the activity). For instance, in introducing rank-ordering, the teacher might preface the activity by saying, "What I'd like us to do now is to take some time to consider alternatives and consequences of our choices, as well as a chance to listen well to others' ideas." Again, it is vital to be aware that the same activity could be used or stretched in different ways to address different objectives and skills. It's up to you!

Bread makes itself, by your kindness, with your help, with imagination running through you, dough under hand, you are breadmaking itself, which is why breadmaking is so fulfilling and rewarding. A recipe doesn't belong to anyone. Given to me, I give it to you. Only a guide, only a skeletal framework. You must fill in the flesh according to your nature and desire. Your life, your love will bring these words into creation. This cannot be taught. You already know. So please, cook, love, feel, create!

THE CONTEXT OF THE ACTIVITIES

We think it is important for teachers to keep in mind that values clarification seeks to look at the "whole person"—thoughts, feelings, actions, interpersonal relationships. Our premise is that if people feel more valuable, they would be less likely to engage in self-destructive behaviors as well as behaviors that might hurt others (e.g. "you don't

[1] Published by special arrangement with Shambhala Publications, Inc., Berkeley, California. From *The Tassajara Bread Book* by Edward Espe Brown. © 1970 by the Chief Priest, Zen Center, San Francisco.

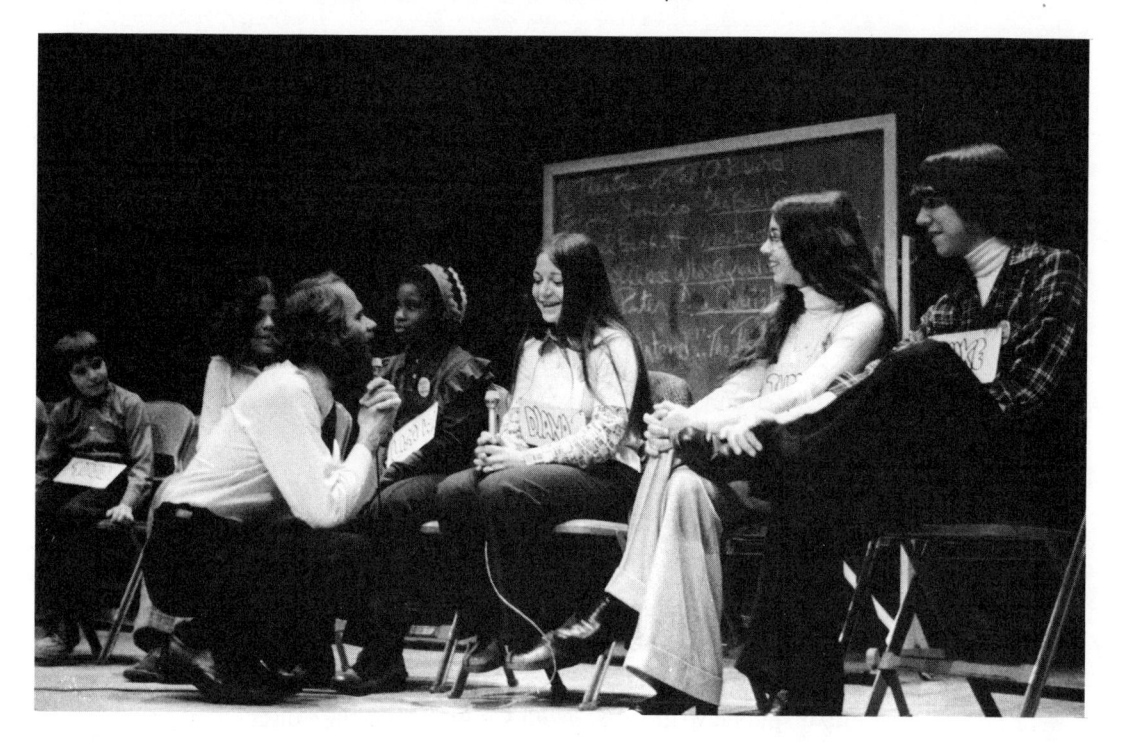

have to blow out my candle to make yours glow brighter"). Following this line of reasoning, we believe that people who feel good about themselves and who have skills in making valuable decisions will be less likely to engage in the abuse of substances (e.g. drugs), or other people.

It is important that the values-clarification activities listed in this chapter be integrated with ways to help students develop better self-concepts,[2] as well as with strategies that focus on other areas of conflict and confusion (e.g. family, friends, work, leisure, future plans, religion, race, politics, money). In other words, we are saying that we can't deal with the "drug problem" (or any "problem") in isolation. We need to help students look at their entire selves, lives, and life styles.

DIRECTIONS FOR THE ACTIVITIES

Just as there are innumerable ways to modify the content of any one valuing activity, there also is an infinite variety of directions that could

---

[2]Jack Canfield and Harold C. Wells, *100 Ways to Enhance Self-Concept in the Classroom* (Englewood Cliffs, N.J.: Prentice-Hall, Inc., 1976); William Purkey, *Self Concept and School Achievement* (Englewood Cliffs, N.J.: Prentice-Hall, Inc., 1970).

be used with any activity. Again, we encourage you to think divergently—and to fit the directions to the purpose you have in mind for the activity, as well as to the readiness level of your students. The material that follows provides skeletal outlines of directions for each of the five activities in this chapter.

Rank-ordering

Here, students are simply asked to make some choices and to identify priorities and preferences. The students rank a set of elements according to a specific dimension. In fact, this is the "formula" for any rank-order: dimension + elements. For example, you might ask your students to rank from 1 to 3:

Dimension: which do you think would be hardest for you to accept in your teenage son:

Elements:

____ to get someone pregnant while not married

____ to be dependent on "hard" drugs

____ to date someone from another race

This ranking could be done privately (in a journal or class diary), and/or publicly (in small groups, in a whole-class discussion, in conference with the teacher).

Values-voting

Here, the teacher presents the students with a series of questions, each one starting with the words: "How many of you . . .?" The students respond by using one of the following hand signals: If they are strongly and fervently in favor of the idea presented, they wave their hands vigorously, with thumbs pointed up; if they are in favor of the idea, they hold their hands steady, with thumbs pointed up; if they are against or don't believe in the idea presented, they hold their thumbs down; if they are violently against the idea, they pump their hands vigorously, with their thumbs pointed down; if they choose to pass on the question, they fold their hands (as in all activities, students have the right "to pass"—this is not questioned).

Some teachers like to use the values-voting activity as an energizer and thought-provoker/seed-planter. Others like to use the questions as a discussion-starter or as an introduction to a unit.

Spread of opinion

This activity is designed to help students see the range of opinions that are possible on any one issue. The teacher identifies the issue at hand, and then draws a line on the board. At either end of the line, the teacher identifies an outrageous extreme—and then asks students to indicate where they stand on the line. This can be facilitated through students recording the spread of opinion in their journals, through small-group discussions, through placing their initials on the line in a whole-group discussion, and/or by literally standing up physically along a line down the middle of the room.

For instance, here's how one spread of opinion line looked in a class taught by one of the authors:

Issue: safety: wearing seat belts

Scissors Stan   *Ron Gail*   *Tom Steve*   *Helen*   Drive-in Dan

Scissors is the kind of person who absolutely detests seat belts—in fact, he'll even go around parking lots with scissors in hand, and cut out all the seat belts he can find. Dan is the kind of person who absolutely swears by seat belts—in fact, he'll even wear them to a drive-in movie, and make sure that both he and his date remain buckled in throughout the movie.

Moral dilemmas There are two kinds of moral-dilemma activities. The first involves the teacher presenting the students with a "What-would-you-do-if . . . ?" situation. Here, the students are asked to generate possible alternatives—to do an alternatives search. The second kind of moral dilemma involves the students hearing a story, and then being asked to do some rank-orders based on the story.

Inventory Here, students are given an opportunity to become "merchants"—to take stock of some of the "shelves" in their lives. The inventory includes the following elements: (1) a listing of items (e.g., 20 things you love to do in life; 15 people who are significant to you; 10 TV shows you watch; 20 items in your medicine cabinet); (2) an analysis of these items through codings (e.g., place a $ next to those things you love to do that cost at least $5); and (3) an opportunity for the student to "process" or draw conclusions/inferences from the data he or she has generated and analyzed (in fact, this step is crucial for *any* valuing activity).

STRATEGIES IN HUMAN SEXUALITY

Rank-orders

1. What is the hardest for you to communicate?
   ___ praise
   ___ disapproval
   ___ hurt

2. What do you look for in a friend?
   ___ someone who is good-looking
   ___ someone who is fun to be with
   ___ someone who gets good grades

3. What kind of massage would you like the most? To give? To receive?
   ___ head
   ___ foot
   ___ back

4. What do you think is the best environment in which to raise a child?
   ___ a nuclear family
   ___ a communal arrangement
   ___ a good boarding school

5. If you were pregnant, and unmarried would you
   ___ get an abortion
   ___ marry someone you didn't love, so the baby would be with the father
   ___ give the baby up for adoption

6. What should we do regarding masturbation?
   ___ allow it, tolerate it
   ___ encourage it
   ___ forbid it

7. What should schools do regarding information on venereal disease?
   ___ not make it available
   ___ insist that every senior should receive information on it
   ___ make it available at a drop-in center

8 Who do you think should be most responsible for birth-control information?

___ the school

___ parents

___ the family doctor

___ friends

9 Presently, who do you see as most influential in disseminating birth-control information to high-school students? (This reflects one way of "stretching" a rank order—using a different question with the same content.)

___ the school

___ parents

___ the family doctor

10 At what age do you think that schools should make birth-control information available to students?

___ not at all

___ elementary school

___ junior high

___ senior high

11 What do you think is most important in sustaining a relationship?

___ a strong sexual bond

___ the couple knows how to fight, be angry, express feelings cleanly

___ the similar cultural backgrounds

12 Which are the most important factors working against a long-term relationship?

___ different economic class

___ incompatible astrological signs

___ bad sexual adjustment

13 What should be our attitude toward people who choose homosexuality?

___ they should be respected

___ they should be put in jail

___ they should be put in a mental institution

14 What does a "hug" mean to you?

___ an expression of love

___ a casual greeting

___ the prelude to seduction

15 What turns you on the most?
- ____ sight
- ____ smell
- ____ touch

16 Which of these would you most like to read?
- ____ *Playboy*
- ____ Masters and Johnson
- ____ *The Joy of Sex*

17 What is most important to you in a future mate?
- ____ someone who is a virgin
- ____ someone who is sexually attractive
- ____ someone who is smarter than you

18 Which of these patterns is most desirable to you?
- ____ coupling with one person for life
- ____ serial monogamy
- ____ staying single
- ____ coupling with one person for life, with affairs on the side

19 When you see a childless couple, how do you usually react?
- ____ "Oh, the poor things."
- ____ "Oh, the lucky things."
- ____ "I bet they're still trying."

20 Which of these would you most want to avoid in a relationship?
- ____ boredom
- ____ no communication
- ____ infidelity

21 Which of these would you most prefer to do?
- ____ make love
- ____ see the Superbowl
- ____ eat a full gourmet meal

43 VALUES CLARIFICATION ACTIVITIES   Chapter 4

22 Which would make you wonder the most about the sex life of a couple you visited?

___ they have a TV in the bedroom

___ they have a bookshelf behind their bed, lined with sexy novels

___ one of the couple spoke about masturbating regularly

23 How would you prefer to meet someone?

___ on the street

___ in class

___ in a singles bar

___ on a blind date

24 How often should couples make love?

___ once a day

___ twice a day

___ three times a week

___ only when they both feel like it

25 How do you see sex?

___ as fun

___ as reward

___ as proof

___ as an adventure

___ as a purely playful activity

___ as an expression of love and caring

Here is some space in which you can generate additional activities . . . your own curriculum-development practicum. You can do it!

VALUES CLARIFICATION ACTIVITIES Chapter 4

Values-voting How many of you:

1. Learned about where babies come from from your parents?
2. Learned where babies come from from other kids on the block?
3. Learned where babies come from from a book?
4. Feel you have enough information about birth control?
5. Feel you have enough information about VD?
6. Feel that school should have an office giving out birth-control information?
7. Think that scaring people is an effective deterrent to VD?
8. Like kissing or hugging scenes in the movies?
9. Think kissing should be banned from TV?
10. Get at least four hugs each day?
11. Give at least four hugs each day?
12. Have seen a dog in heat?
13. Have seen a pet give birth?
14. Have a pet that gets more physical affection than some people in the house?
15. Have seen an X-rated film?
16. Would like to see an X-rated film?
17. Are positive that you could not appear in an X-rated film?
18. Have been told that awful things would happen to you if you masturbated?
19. Think sex education belongs only in the home?
20. Know someone who had to get married because she was pregnant?
21. Think pregnant girls should be allowed to attend school?
22. Would have your parents' support in obtaining birth control methods?
23. Would not be able to tell your parents you were having intercourse?
24. Think boys should be able to cry in public without ridicule?
25. Want someone who has more sexual experience than you as a husband/wife?
26. Would want to take a course in proper "intercourse technique"?
27. Would like to teach a course in proper "intercourse technique"?
28. Have read books by Masters and Johnson?
29. Have read *The Joy of Sex*?
30. Read *Playboy* regularly?
31. Think that marrying a virgin is desirable?
32. Think parents should not walk around naked in front of their children?
33. Think parents should not walk around naked in front of their children after the children have started going to school?
34. Think college-dormitory bathrooms should be coed?
35. Close and lock the door when you go to the toilet?
36. Don't mind someone brushing their teeth while you're on the toilet?
37. Support the slogan, "Save water, shower with a friend"?
38. Think it is O.K. to have a boy/girl friend when you're in first grade?
39. Would not be interested in developing a relationship with someone who is divorced?
40. See divorce as failure?
41. Feel that marriage is forever?
42. Would consider a trial marriage of one year or longer?

43 Think it's O.K. to have two boy/girl friends at once?
44 Are committed to monogamy?
45 Think you could handle an "open marriage"?
46 Are free of jealousy?
47 Think there is a double standard?
48 Think that a great amount of sexual experience before marriage is important?
49 Are convinced that women can get as much pleasure from sex as men?
50 Have seen a movie where two people didn't live happily ever after (without death intervening)?
51 Know of at least one "perfect" marriage?
52 Would stay together (rather than get divorced) for the sake of the children?
53 Think you could identify the secret of that perfect marriage?
54 Would like to have a perfect marriage?
55 Think mates should be changed every few years (serial monogamy)?
56 Think you may remain single?
57 Will have at least two kids if you choose to have children?
58 Think a wife should keep her maiden name?
59 Think people should have to get a license in order to become parents?
60 Feel that making love is not successful if both don't reach orgasm every time?
61 Will not have children if you marry?
62 Will have children even if you aren't married?
63 Would feel satisfied if either or both partners reached orgasm half the time?
64 Feel the focus on orgasm is overdone?
65 Feel it's okay for married couples to masturbate?
66 Think using a computer is a good way to meet someone?
67 Would go on a blind date?
68 Can handle singles bars?
69 Enjoy mixers (e.g. at college)?
70 Would consider having a nude massage with friends?
71 Would be interested in experimenting with sex outdoors?
72 See a difference between "having sex" and "making love"?
73 Have ever gone skinny dipping?
74 Would be scared to have sex with someone much older than you?
75 Would consider having intercourse with someone of another race?

VALUES CLARIFICATION ACTIVITIES   Chapter 4

Here is some space in which you can generate additional activities . . . your own curriculum-development practicum. You can do it!

Spread of opinion

1. Under-the-covers Cal ———————————————— Out-in-the-open Oliver

   Oliver thinks that information about VD should be disseminated to children in elementary school, with graphic descriptions and pictures. Cal feels that you'd just be opening a Pandora's box if you told children about VD, and, besides, VD is "dirty."

2. Auto-erotic Eric ———————————————————— Warty Walter

   Eric drives himself to the heights of ecstasy every chance he gets, reasoning that he has to love himself first before he can love anyone else. Walter is so turned off by masturbation that he severely punishes his own children whenever he catches them scratching their crotches.

3. Gloves Gladys ———————————————————— Mattress Milly

   Regarding premarital intercourse, Gladys will have no part of it, and loudly condemns anyone even considering it. Milly believes that one needs to experiment fully before marriage in order to make a wise choice—she thinks it's fine even on a first date.

4. No-nuke Ned ————————————————————— Core Carl

   Concerning the viability of the nuclear family, Ned believes that its time has passed—he feels that anything is better than having children growing up in a nuclear family, even if it means sending them to boarding school at the age of three. Carl sees the nuclear family as the core of his life and believes that there is no other place where children can find the intimacy that the nuclear family offers.

5. Touchy-feely Fred ———————————————————— Iron Mike

   When it comes to touching, Fred is very comfortable—when first meeting someone (of either sex), he will warmly greet them with a big hug and kiss. Mike never allows himself to touch or be touched—even by his intimates; if an accident occurs, and Mike is touched, he will quickly run and wash the spot where the touch occurred.

6. Ultimate Olga ———————————————— Easy-come, easy-go Gertrude

   When it comes to orgasm, Olga thinks it's essential to any good relationship—so essential that she thinks both partners ought to climax each time they make love, or else the relationship is a failure. Gertrude takes an easy-come, easy-go attitude regarding orgasm—it's nice when it happens, but it's no sweat when it doesn't.

7. Size-'em-up Sam ———————————————————— No-see Cyrano

   As far as "looks" are concerned, Sam is the kind of guy who rates every woman he sees on a ten-point scale, and won't go out on a date with any woman who rates less than a "seven". Cyrano is the kind of guy to whom looks are totally unimportant—he even feels that people should put on blindfolds when they go out on dates.

49 VALUES CLARIFICATION ACTIVITIES Chapter 4

8 All-in-the-family Frank ———————————— One-on-one Juan

Frank believes that marriages should be wide open—that both partners feel free to "play around"; Swinger is his middle name. Juan cherishes the sanctity of marriage to the point where he would immediately divorce his wife if he found out that she even touched another man.

Here is some space in which you can generate additional activities . . . your own curriculum-development practicum. You can do it!

Moral dilemmas

1. What would you do if your best friend, John, asked you to keep a secret—that he has VD—and you know that John is going out with another of your friends, Joan?
2. What would you do if you have a date with a boy/girl you aren't too wild about, and an old flame comes by just before you leave; would you keep the date?
3. What would you do if you are a parent and you walk into your son/daughter's room while he/she is masturbating?
4. What would you do if your daughter dropped her purse and some birth-control pills fell out?
5. What would you do if your son/daughter "hangs around" with a promiscuous crowd, and he/she wants to have a party at your house on a weekend when you'll be away?
6. What would you do if your parents won't allow you to go to parties where there are boys and girls (and you know you could lie to them)?
7. What would you do if you're having a pajama party and know that some boys will probably "crash" it—how would you dress?
8. What would you do if you had just broken up with your boy/girlfriend and he/she started going out with your best friend?
9. What would you do if you knew that a student at school was selling fake birth-control pills?
10. What would you do if you wanted to show caring for another person?
11. What would you do if you wanted to send love long distance?
12. What would you do if you would like to go out with a particular boy/girl, but know your friends disapprove of him/her?
13. What would you do if you would like to go out with a particular boy/girl but know your parents disapprove of him/her?
14. What would you do if you had a chance to borrow an older friend's ID card and go to a pick-up bar?
15. What would you do if two of your best friends were engaged to be married, and you didn't think they were "made" for each other?
16. What would you do if your best friend had just broken up with his boy/girlfriend, and really needed support?
17. What would you do if you needed some caring?
18. What would you do if you were feeling angry?
19. What would you do if you wanted to celebrate?
20. What kind of ceremony would you want if you were getting married?
21. What would you do if your date wanted to kiss you the first time you went out?

As mentioned at the beginning of this chapter, there is another kind of moral-dilemma strategy: The teacher (or a student) presents a story chock-full of values issues, and then the students are asked to do a rank-order based on the story. This individual ranking can be followed by a whole-class discussion and/or by challenging the students to reach consensus on their rankings in small discussion groups.

Here are some sample stories that you might want to use or adapt to the particular group with whom you're working:

51 VALUES CLARIFICATION ACTIVITIES   Chapter 4

22   Gail, a high-school senior, has been going steady with Jeff for a year and a half. She and Jeff have recently decided that they would like to have intercourse, and Jeff refuses to use a condom, because he claims it will reduce his pleasure. So, Gail goes to her best friend, Alice, to ask for information about where and how she can get the Pill. Alice is furious with Gail, calls her a slut, and refuses to give her any information. The next day, Gail asks her most trusted teacher at school the same question—and the teacher, Miss Green, agrees to obtain some pills for her. Several weeks later, Gail's parents discover the pills in her bureau, and demand that she reveal how she got them. Gail is scared and honest as she tells of Miss Green's involvement. Her parents are outraged, go to the school board, and eventually have Miss Green fired.

In your estimation, who was the most responsible person in this story? Rank them in order.

_____ Gail

_____ Jeff

_____ Alice

_____ Miss Green

_____ Gail's parents

23   Once upon a time, there was a river that was practically overflowing with alligators. As you may have guessed, it was called Alligator River. A girl named Abigail lived on the west bank of the river. Her boy friend, Greg, lived on the opposite bank. Abigail and Greg were very much in love with each other and wanted very much to see each other. But there was one slight complication: no boat, and an alligator-filled river stood between them. Abigail decided to seek help so that she could see her boy friend, Greg. She approached Sinbad the Sailor, who, as his name might indicate, owned a boat. Now this was very fortunate for Abigail, because Sinbad's boat was exactly what she needed to get across the river. She explained her situation to Sinbad and asked if she could borrow his boat. Sinbad thought for a moment and then replied: "Sure, you can borrow my boat, but only under one condition. The condition is that you sleep with me tonight." This startled Abigail, because she didn't want to sleep with Sinbad; she just wanted to borrow his boat so she could see Greg. So, she told Sinbad to forget it, and wandered off seeking someone else who would help her.

After a great deal of time, Abigail was unable to find anyone else who could aid her. Discouraged, she returned home, where she sought out her mother. Explaining her dilemma and Sinbad's proposition, Abigail asked her mother about what she should do. Mom responded with: "Look, Abigail, you're a big girl now; it's about time you started making these kinds of decisions for yourself." With that, Mom turned and walked away.

Abigail thought and thought. Finally, she decided to take Sinbad up on his offer, because she wanted to see Greg so very much. So, that night

Abigail and Sinbad slept with each other. The next morning, Sinbad, true to his word, lent his boat to Abigail. Abigail sailed across the river and saw her beloved. After spending a few delightful hours together, Abigail felt compelled to tell Greg what had happened. After she had related her whole story, Greg blew up completely: "You what? I can't believe you did that! I—I can't believe you slept with him! That's it. It's all over. Just forget the relationship. Get out of my life!"

Distraught, Abigail wandered off. She came upon a fellow named Slug. Borrowing his shoulder to shed her tears, Abigail related her tale to Slug. Slug then went looking for Greg (with Abigail close behind). Slug found Greg and proceeded to beat the stuffing out of him, with Abigail standing there, laughing.[3]

In your estimation, who was the most admirable person in this story? Rank them in order.

____ Abigail

____ Greg

____ Sinbad

____ Mom

____ Slug

24 The following people have applied to be on the school system's advisory group on sex education. Whom would you choose to fill the five slots on the committee? Rank them in order.

   ____ A forty-year-old male violinist who is a suspected narcotics pusher

   ____ A thirty-four-year-old male architect who is thought to be homosexual

   ____ A twenty-six-year-old lawyer

   ____ The lawyer's twenty-four-year-old wife (They both want to be on the committee together, thinking it important to have a husband-wife couple on the group; rumor has it that they've had some marital difficulties.)

   ____ A seventy-five-year-old priest

   ____ A thirty-four-year-old retired prostitute who was so successful that she's been living off her annuities for five years

   ____ A twenty-year-old Black militant

   ____ A twenty-three-year-old-female graduate student who speaks publicly on the virtues of chastity

[3]For another version of this story, see Joel Goodman and Laurie Hawkins, "Value Clarification: Meeting a Challenge in Education," *Colloquy*, 5, no. 5 (May 1972): 18-22.

53 VALUES CLARIFICATION ACTIVITIES Chapter 4

___ A thirty-nine-year-old female M.D. who is an avowed bigot

___ An elementary-school boy

___ A high-school student who is very unpopular with peers[4]

25 Pam met Fred at high school. On their first date, they really had fun, and the same on their second date. As a matter of fact, they began to see each other a lot, for they really could relax together, study together, do most anything together.

It was on their third date, in front of the fireplace in Pam's basement play room one night when her parents weren't home, that Fred first declared he loved Pam and never wanted to be without her. The setting was perfect—the warm, flickering fire, parents gone, beautifully spoken words of love. Pam gave in to Fred quite easily—the second "I love you" did it.

It wasn't long until Pam began talking about when they'd get married, the number of kids they'd have, and so on. She was so busy planning their life together that she wasn't aware of Fred's changing attitude and restlessness.

It was at about this time that Pam had her yearly checkup, something her mother always insisted upon for all her children. The blood test showed it—Pam had syphillis. Yes, she had contacted that thing called VD. At first she didn't believe it because she felt fine. How could she have a disease when she felt fine? The doctor convinced her that yes, it was possible.

Pam went deep into thought . . . but that's got to be Fred. And we're going together. How could he have gotten it? How could this be happening to me?

The doctor told Pam's mother against her wishes. Pam's mother, in a rage, beat her, saying she deserved no better, as she'd disgraced the family. She grounded Pam for three solid months, and to top it off, absolutely forbade Pam to see Fred again. Pam (sneaking around it) confronted Fred at school. He admitted to seeing another girl a few times as pressure from Pam had gotten stronger and stronger. Yes, he knew he had VD; he could tell, but he figured it was Pam's responsibility. If she hadn't pressured him, it never would have happened in the first place.[5]

In your estimation, who was the most responsible person in this story? Rank them in order.

___ Pam

___ Fred

___ Doctor

___ Mother

[4]These characters were borrowed from Joel B. Goodman's "An Application of Values Clarification to the Teaching of Psychology," *Periodically*, 31 March, 1972, p. 4.

[5]This story was generated by Margie Ingram.

Here is some space in which you can generate additional activities . . . your own curriculum-development practicum. You can do it!

Inventories

1 *All the people you've kissed*

    S All the people you had/have sexual feelings for.
    A You consider the person to be an acquaintance.
    F You consider the person to be a friend.
    X You haven't seen that person in five years.
    O The person is much older than you.
    ***** Five people whose kisses have meant the most to you.

Thought questions:

1 What does a kiss mean to you?
2 What else can you do in addition to kissing to touch another person's life?
3 Would you agree with the notion that "kisses are sweeter than wine"?

2 *People to whom you are attracted*

    S Same sex as you.
    M Mutual attraction.
    P Physical attraction.
    I Common interests, values.
    C You've developed a close relationship with that person.
    T You feel you can trust that person.

Thought questions:

1 What in yourself do you find attractive? What do others find attractive about you?
2 Can you think of any ways in which you can make yourself more attractive? Is that important to you?
3 What is it in other people that attracts you on a first-impression basis? On a long-term basis?

3 *"Old wives' tales" you've heard about masturbation; contraception*

    P   You first heard it in preadolescence.
    F   You learned it from your friends.
    M/D You learned it from your parents.
    I   You wish you had more information on it.
    B   You still believe it, at least in part.

Thought questions:

1 Who was the most significant influence on your developing attitudes related to sexuality?
2 How did/do you deal with conflicting information from your friends, your parents, your own experience?
3 To whom would you go now if you had a question related to sexuality? What might hold you back from approaching that person with your question?

4 *Qualities of an ideal mate*

- **M** Your mother has this quality.
- **F** Your father has this quality.
- **+** You have this quality.
- ***** You would like to develop this quality further.
- **B** You think that it is essential for both partners in the relationship to have this quality.
- **I** The five most important qualities.

Thought questions:

1 I am proud that I . . .
2 What suggestions would you make to someone who wanted to develop a particular quality (pick one from your list)?
3 Where do you draw the line between accepting a person as he/she is, and pushing/nudging that person to grow?

5 *Rules (stated or unstated) that govern your sexual behavior when with a significant other person*

- **X** You wish the rule didn't exist; you would like to change it.
- **I** You initiated the rule.
- **6** You hope this rule will still be in effect six months from now.
- **P** Your parents have this rule in their relationship.
- **O** You've had this rule in other relationships.

Thought questions:

1 How do you think people should go about "making rules" in relationships? What do you do when you and the other person disagree about the "rules"?
2 What can you do to maintain a rule ("6" coding)? What can you do to change a rule?
3 Which three rules do you think are the most basic for any intimate relationship?

6 *The qualities of the best marriage you know*

- **I** You identify with.
- ***** Something you would like to get better at.
- **L** A "learnable" quality—not just occurring by chance.
- **R** Involves some element of risk.
- **+** The three most important qualities at the foundation of the relationship.

Thought questions:

1 For you, what part does "risk" play in a relationship? Do you want to risk more or risk less in your present relationships?

57 VALUES CLARIFICATION ACTIVITIES Chapter 4

2 If you could ask the two people in the best marriage you know only one question, what would it be?
3 Can you describe/role play how this couple would handle a disagreement? How would you handle disagreements in a relationship?

7 *Books you've read that had explicit sex in them*

- C You read it cover to cover.
- M You would see the movie.
- 6 You think it would be okay for a six-year-old to read it.
- T It taught you something about your sexual behavior.
- C It confused your attitudes.
- I You identified with it.

Thought questions:

1 For the book that you read cover to cover, what was it about it that grabbed you?
2 If you were to write a book with explicit sex in it—perhaps a manual—what would you title it?
3 What would be the consequences of having a six-year-old read a book with explicit sex in it? What would be the consequences of hiding that book from the six-year-old?

8 *TV shows or commercials that have explicit or implicit messages about sexuality*

- E Explicit.
- I Implicit.
- A You agree with the message.
- in It has influenced your sexual attitudes.
- S You consider the message to be sexist.
- C You hope your children will learn this message.

Thought questions:

1 Write a motto for the two messages with which you agree the most. Write a motto for the two messages with which you disagree the most.
2 For you, what are the elements of a "sexist" message?
3 If you could send one message about sexuality to people all across the country, what would it be? What kind of commercial could you develop that would reflect that message?

9 *Ways one person can "touch" another*

- I You like to be touched in this way.
- T You like to touch others in this way.
- P Your parents touched you in this way while you were growing up.
- R Involves some element of risk.
- 65 You still hope to be touched in this way when you're sixty-five.
- 1 You think people need to be touched this way at least once a day.

Thought questions:

1 Can you recall a very touching moment in your life? What made it so touching?
2 In general, do you see yourself as an initiator or receiver of touch? Are you happy with this pattern? Is there anything you want to do about it?
3 If a detective came across your inventory, what conclusions could he or she draw about you?

10 *A boy is . . . a girl is . . .*

    I   *You identify with this quality or trait.*
    T   *You think this is true for all boys/girls.*
    S   *You consider this to be a stereotype.*
    C   *You think this quality or trait is learned through conditioning.*

Thought questions:

1 Make a collage that reflects your response to "A boy is . . ." Make another collage that reflects your response to "A girl is . . ." Do you think people could identify which is which?
2 Is there any difference between "masculine" and "feminine"? If so, how would you describe it?
3 What recommendations wuld you have for someone who wanted to stop stereotyping people?

11 *Boys can . . . girls can . . .*

    I   *You identify with this.*
    T   *You think this is true for all boys/girls.*
    S   *You consider this to be stereotype.*
    C   *You think this is learned through conditioning.*

Thought questions:

1 Play the song, "Parents Are People," from the record "Free to Be You and Me." What is the message of the song? Do you agree or disagree with it?
2 Is there anything you think that boys/girls can't do?
3 Name one goal that you have for yourself. What might get in the way of your achieving that goal? Is there anything you can do to overcome that obstacle(s)?

12 *Boys shouldn't . . . girls shouldn't . . .*

    I   *You identify with this.*
    T   *You think this is true for all boys/girls.*
    C   *You think this is learned through conditioning.*
    P   *You learned this from your parents.*
    D   *You disagree with this.*

VALUES CLARIFICATION ACTIVITIES Chapter 4

Thought questions:

1. If you were a parent, what kinds of "shouldn't" guidelines would you try to teach your children? How might you go about teaching them?
2. What do you see as your own strengths? What do you see as your own limits? Can you see any way of using your strengths to stretch your limits?
3. What would happen to a person if he/she went through life totally contradicting each of the items in your inventory?

Here is some space in which you can generate additional activities . . . your own curriculum-development practicum. You can do it!

STRATEGIES IN DRUG EDUCATION

Rank orders

1. Which of these do you consider to be most harmful?

    ____ Two drinks before dinner every night

    ____ Smoking pot once a week

    ____ Smoking a pack of cigarettes every day

2. Which of the following would you least like your children to do?

    ____ Drinking two beers before dinner every night

    ____ Smoking pot twice a week

    ____ Smoking a pack of cigarettes a day

3. Which of these are you least likely to try?

    ____ LSD

    ____ Cigarette smoking

    ____ Drinking cocktails

4. What do you think is the most effective way to discourage drug abuse?

    ____ Horror stories from exaddicts

    ____ Horror stories from policemen

    ____ Factual information about the effects of drugs

5. If a friend were using LSD, which would you do?

    ____ Report him/her

    ____ Join him; go along with the crowd

    ____ Avoid him/her

    ____ Ask him/her to stop

6. If your son or daughter were smoking pot, which would you do?

    ____ Report him/her to the authorities

    ____ Ground him/her for two weeks

    ____ Ignore it?

    ____ Talk with him/her about it

7. If a parent were smoking heavily, how might you get him/her to stop?

    ____ Send a letter saying how much you love him/her

    ____ Leave the room whenever he/she smokes

    ____ Hide his/her cigarettes

8 What might attract you to the use of drugs?

____ The chance to expand your consciousness

____ The need to go along with the crowd

____ Curiosity

____ The desire to escape boredom

____ A wish for excitement, thrills

____ The need to relax

9 If you came across someone pushing drugs to elementary school students, which would you do?

____ Report him/her

____ Ignore it

____ Tell the students to stay away

10 Which of these facts would discourage you from using alcohol?

____ An alcoholic's life span is shortened by ten to 12 years

____ In half the murders in the United States, either the killer or the victim, or both, have been drinking

____ Alcohol costs $15 billion per year in the United States just in terms of time lost from work

11 In your home, what is your attitude toward drugs?

____ Total abstinence

____ Laissez-faire

____ Parents encourage the children to try alcohol (and praise their ability to hold their liquor)

12 How do you perceive alcohol?

____ As a socializer

____ As a tranquilizer

____ As a depressant

13 Which do you prefer?

____ Beer

____ Wine

____ Hard liquor

____ Milk

14 What would you rely on if you needed help in breaking a habit?

    ____ Self-discipline

    ____ Talking with a friend

    ____ Talking with your doctor

15 If you were a senator voting on how to allocate $1 million, what would be your priorities?

    ____ Drug-abuse educational programs

    ____ Drug-counseling crisis centers

    ____ Long-term drug-rehabilitation centers

16 Through which of these would you prefer to expand your consciousness?

    ____ Meditation

    ____ Pot

    ____ Reading

17 What is the best way to "control" drug abuse?

    ____ Decriminalization

    ____ Harsh penalties

    ____ Educational programs

18 Regarding drugs, to whom would you be most likely to listen?

    ____ An exaddict

    ____ A physician

    ____ A policeman

    ____ Peers

19 Which of these is your position?

    ____ There is no drug abuse problem

    ____ Legal drugs are abused

    ____ Illegal drugs are abused

20 Regarding drugs, which of the following would be your motto?

    ____ "Curiosity killed the cat"

    ____ "Try it, you'll like it"

    ____ "I'd rather fight than switch"

    ____ "You only go around once in life—get all the gusto you can"

VALUES CLARIFICATION ACTIVITIES Chapter 4

21 Which of these do you consider to be most harmful?

___ A parent with a violent temper

___ A parent who is an alcoholic

___ A family in which there is no love between the parents

22 What do you think our country's priorities should be?

___ Drug education

___ Ecology

___ Poverty

23 Who do you think should be responsible for drug education?

___ The family doctor

___ The home

___ The school

Here is some space in which you can generate additional activities . . . your own curriculum-development practicum. You can do it!

Voting questions   How many of you:

1 Think there should be a minimum age for drinking?
2 Think that the minimum drinking age should be fifteen? Eighteen? Twenty-one?
3 Think there should be a minimum age for smoking?
4 Think that marijuana should be decriminalized?
5 Have ever faked your age in order to get a drink?
6 Know someone who is hooked on alcohol? On cigarettes?
7 Have tried to talk with that person?
8 Think smoking should be banned in public places?
9 Have ever driven after drinking?
10 Have "quit smoking" at least once?
11 Would like to stop smoking?
12 Think you'll smoke or drink when you're older?
13 Hope your children won't smoke or drink?
14 Have ever considered putting up a no-smoking sign in your house?
15 Offer guests a drink in your home?
16 Have ever gone bar-hopping?
17 Take aspirin when you have a headache?
18 Drink at least two cups of coffee each morning?
19 Have ever had a hangover?
20 Think restaurants should have smoking and nonsmoking sections?
21 Drink or smoke more now than you did three years ago?
22 Get drunk at least once a month?
23 Consider alcohol to be a drug?
24 Would consider using a sleeping pill?
25 Take novocaine when you go to the dentist?
26 Enjoy taking such medicines as cough syrup?
27 Think doctors are too drug-oriented?
28 Think that the society was right in passing Prohibition laws?
29 Think teachers should have the right to search students' lockers?
30 Smoke cigarettes and enjoy it?

Here is some space in which you can generate additional activities . . . your own curriculum-development practicum. You can do it!

67 VALUES CLARIFICATION ACTIVITIES   Chapter 4

Spread of opinion

1   Band-Aid Bill ———————————————————— Futuristic Frank

Bill is the kind of person who thinks that we need to solve the drug problem *now*, that our children's lives are too precious to play around with; he advocates stringent antidrug measures immediately. Frank is the kind of person who believes in the effectiveness of a long-term program that will deal not only with symptoms but with causes. Although there may not be any immediately observable benefits from Frank's approach, he feels that it is in the best interests of people.

2   Stoned Steve ———————————————————————— Pure Paul

Steve is always high on one drug or another. He begins his morning by popping a couple of pills, sneaks some cigarettes in the bathroom during school, smokes some grass after school with his friends, and ends his day by taking some sleeping pills. Paul is so antidrug that he will refuse to take even an aspirin when he has a splitting headache. He avoids coffee and tea, because of the caffein in them, and condemns the weakness in people who need to rely on them.

3   Natural-high Helen ——————————————— Ecstasy-machine Mary

Helen likes to feel high, but she insists on getting there through "natural" processes. She believes that all the ingredients for "highness" are found within herself, nature, and her friends. Mary, on the other hand, thinks that we should make use of our technological advances to create pleasure for people; all kinds of mechanical and chemical devices are within bounds for her.

4   Risky Rhoda ———————————————————————— Cautious Carla

When it comes to risk taking, Rhoda lives by the old carpe-diem theme: Play today, for tomorrow we may die. She will try anything once, her curiosity being insatiable; she's never been known to turn down a dare. Carla is so timid that she will never try anything unless she is absolutely assured of the outcome. Before buying anything, she checks to see that the Food and Drug Administration, the Department of Health, Education and Welfare, and Ralph Nader all vouch for its safety.

5   Free-will Walter ——————————————————— Prohibition Peter

When it comes to cigarette smoking, Walter just can't get enough of it. He loves the smell and taste of tobacco, and especially loves to be in an elevator filled with cigarette, pipe, and cigar smoke. He is ardently against any regulations of smoking in public places. Peter is so allergic to smoke that he will often suffer an asthma attack at the sight of a lit cigarette. Peter, in fact, is so antismoking that he goes around and places out-of-order signs on cigarette machines, and will spit in the face of anyone lighting up in public.

Here is some space in which you can generate additional activities . . . your own curriculum-development practicum. You can do it!

Moral dilemmas

1. What would you do if you saw a fifteen-year-old drinking on his way to school?
2. What would you do if you saw a fifteen-year-old drinking on her way to school?
3. What would you do if you came across some students smoking cigarettes in the lavatory?
4. What would you do if you came across some students smoking pot in the lavatory?
5. What would you do if a person lit up a cigarette in an elevator?
6. What would you do if a person lit up a cigarette in an elevator in which a no-smoking sign was posted?
7. What would you do if your younger brother asked you to get him some liquor?
8. What would you do if your employee came to work drunk?
9. What would you do if a man came up to you on the street and asked you for twenty-five cents for a cup of coffee?
10. What would you do if a person asked you at dinner, "Do you mind if I smoke"?
11. What would you do if you saw a person lying drunk in the gutter?
12. What would you do if you came across a person on a "bum" trip?
13. What would you do if your parents were not home, and your friends urged you to take some of their alcohol for a bash?
14. What would you do if you were asked to serve on your school's drug-education committee?
15. What would you do if you wanted to get a loved one to stop smoking?
16. What would you do if one of your friend's parents were an alcoholic?
17. What would you do if a good friend of yours had been drinking a lot lately?
18. What would you do if a friend, who is drunk, states that he/she will be more than glad to give you a lift home?
19. What would you do if on your first night out together, your date gets totally drunk?
20. What would you do if you are invited to a big weekend bash and someone suggests that "We all get good and drunk!"?
21. What would you do if someone whom you respect and like tells you that he/she feels you have a drinking problem?
22. What would you do if your six-year-old child asks if he/she could have a drink of wine that has been served at dinner?
23. What would you do if the police picked you up for drinking while driving?
24. What would you do if you smelled alcohol on the breath of one of your friends at school?

Another kind of moral dilemma could be presented to students through another version of the Alligator River story. For example, Sinbad's proposition to Abigail could be: "Sure, you can borrow my boat, if you smoke some pot with me." Or, it could be: "Sure . . . if you sell some pot for me." With the rest of the tale remaining constant, this could help the students to grapple with values issues related to drugs.

Here is some space in which you can generate additional activities . . . your own curriculum-development practicum. You can do it!

71 VALUES CLARIFICATION ACTIVITIES Chapter 4

Inventories

1 *Drugs you have seen on TV commercials*

- **$**   Costs at least $3.
- **H**   You have it in your home.
- **T**   You have taken it in the past.
- **F**   You are considering taking it in the future.
- **P**   To be taken to relieve pain.
- **R**   To be taken to relax you.

Thought questions:

1 What are all the ways you can think of to relieve pain?
2 What are some of the things you do in your life to relax?
3 What is your opinion of TV commercials involving drugs? Would you let your own child watch these commercials?

2 *What is in your medicine cabinet at home?*

- **P**   Prescription drugs.
- **S**   Has side-effects.
- **365** Has been in the cabinet for at least a year.
- **T**   You've seen it advertised on TV.
- **F**   Your friends use this drug.
- **I**   You use this only when you have a particular illness.

Thought questions:

1 In considering whether or when to use a particular drug, what effect do the drug's side-effects have in your decision? Do you ever ask your doctor about the side-effects of your prescriptions?
2 If you were to clean out your medicine cabinet, which five items would be the first to go? Which five would be the last to go?
3 Do you see any pattern to the items in your cabinet?

3 *Ways you get "high"*

- **A**   You usually do it alone.
- **P**   You usually do it with another person(s).
- **I**   It is illegal.
- **R**   It involves some risk.
- **N**   It involves "Mommy Nature."
- **W**   You do it at least once each week.

Thought questions:

1 Check out your list with another person. Are there some other ways of "getting high" that you might consider?
2 What are the consequences of each of your ways of getting high? How does each way serve you? What does it cost you?
3 If you were to write a self-contract about ways to get high on life, what would it look like? I will . . . or I hope to . . .

4 *Ways of getting a loved one to stop smoking*

- **T** You've tried in the past and it didn't work.
- **S** You've tried in the past, and it was successful.
- **R** It involves some risk for you (e.g. loss of affection, or disapproval).
- **L** You think this way would have a good chance for a long-lasting effect.
- **Y** You would feel good if someone did this for or to you.

Thought questions:

1. If a loved one were smoking, would you see your intervention as "butting in" or as an act of caring?
2. Have you ever tried to break a habit? What helped you to do it, and what got in your way?
3. If you were trying to break a habit, what kind of support or help might you ask of your friends?

5 *Ways of dealing with stress and distress*

- **D** It involves the use of some drug.
- **T** It involves talking with another person.
- **C** It involves getting it off your chest by crying or laughing.
- **B** You get busier and busier, so that there's no time to think about it.
- **F** Your friends seem to deal with stress and distress in this manner.
- ***** The three ways on your list that seem to work well for you.

Thought questions:

1. If your best friend was facing stress and/or was distressed, what might you do?
2. Can you recall a distressing experience that you handled very well?
3. What is your reaction to the notion that "big boys don't cry"?

Here is some space in which you can generate additional activities . . . your own curriculum-development practicum. You can do it!

STRATEGIES IN NUTRITION EDUCATION

Rank-orders

1. Which of these desserts is your favorite?
   ____ Chocolate pudding
   ____ Fresh pineapple
   ____ Marshmallow cookies

2. Which do you worry about the most?
   ____ Excess of coffee
   ____ Excess of fried foods
   ____ Excess of sugar-laden foods

3. Which diet is your preference?
   ____ All vegetables
   ____ All fruits
   ____ All meat

4. What would motivate you to fast one day each week?
   ____ It develops self-control
   ____ It cleans out your system
   ____ It makes less work, especially cooking
   ____ It cuts down on your food bill

5. Which would you prefer?
   ____ Eating five small meals each day
   ____ Eating two big meals each day
   ____ Eating one big meal and many snacks each day

6. Which of these threatens you the most?
   ____ Seeing people spend money on junk foods
   ____ Seeing people spend money on TV dinners
   ____ Seeing people spend money on packaged cookies
   ____ Seeing people spend money on meat

7. Do you wish that the person(s) who cooks at your home would do any of these?
   ____ Boil vegetables less vigorously
   ____ Fry foods less often
   ____ Serve more raw foods

8 When company comes to dinner, do you do any of these?

___ Serve expensive cuts of meat

___ Serve an abundance of less expensive foods

___ Suggest a pot-luck, bring-your-own format

9 Which of these, in your opinion, is the most healthful "eating out" food?

___ A sundae

___ Pizza

___ A hamburger and French fries

10 Whom do you believe the most when it comes to nutrition?

___ Parents

___ The school nurse

___ TV commercials

11 If you were in the wilderness, would you be likely to eat any of these?

___ Wild berries

___ Canned foods that you had in your knapsack

___ Rabbits you shot

12 For the lowest-cost, best food value, what do you think is the best bargain?

___ Frozen pot pie

___ Canned spaghetti

___ Cottage cheese

13 Which would you like to see the cafeteria serve more often?

___ Frozen spinach

___ Ice cream sandwiches

___ Bean sprouts

14 Which would you most want to control in your own child's eating? If the child were five years old? If the child were fifteen?

___ Popsicles

___ Oreo cookies

___ Baseball bubble gum

15 Which would you most want to control in your own child's drinking?

___ Kool-Aid

___ Wine

___ Coffee

16 If you wanted to lose weight, which of these would you avoid?

   ____ Excess desserts

   ____ Bread

   ____ Potatoes

   ____ Snacks (candy, potato chips, and so on)

17 Would it be hardest for you to live in a family that served which of these?

   ____ Only foods from your own ethnic background

   ____ Meat and potatoes every night

   ____ Only salad plates

Here is some space in which you can generate additional activities . . . your own curriculum-development practicum. You can do it!

Values-voting   How many of you:

1 Drink three glasses of milk each day?
2 Believe the American Dairy Association's assertion that three glasses are necessary?
3 Know someone with a cholesterol problem?
4 Would quit eating eggs if you had a cholesterol problem?
5 Are—or are moving toward being—a vegetarian?
6 Have ever fasted?
7 Use potato chips as a binge food?
8 Have trouble walking past a bakery without buying something?
9 Could work in a candy store and not eat anything there?
10 Come from a "meat-and-potatoes" family?
11 Consistently drink diet soda?
12 Take a daily multivitamin?
13 Feel as if you have tired blood?
14 Wouldn't mind at least one meal each day in pill form?
15 Have in mind a food you would not eat?
16 Know the basic food categories?
17 Were made to clean your plate—or no dessert?
18 Eat dessert before the main dish?
19 Would be happy just living on fruit?
20 Make your own granola?
21 Feel there's a world hunger problem?
22 Who think there's a world hunger problem have changed your habits?
23 See constipation as related to diet?
24 Come from a family where you steamed (instead of boiled) vegetables?
25 Like corn on the cob barely cooked?
26 Like meat rare?
27 Read the ingredients of the food packages you buy?
28 Ever had food poisoning?
29 Come from a family that tends to be trim?
30 Ever felt you had a weight problem?
31 Ever gone on a diet?
32 Ever gone off a diet?
33 Would like to plan the menus for your family?
34 Would rather pack a lunch than buy one at the school cafeteria?
35 Avoid quick-food places and hamburger take-outs?
36 Enjoy midnight snacks?
37 Don't use monosodium glutamate?
38 Snack between meals?
39 Skimp on breakfast?
40 Would rather lose fifteen minutes sleep in order to have a better breakfast?
41 Are thinking of giving up coffee?
42 Refuse to buy food from an automatic vending machine?
43 Like raw vegetables?
44 Are willing to try new foods?

79 VALUES CLARIFICATION ACTIVITIES Chapter 4

45 Avoid fried foods?
46 Could live a week on brown rice and sprouts?
47 Have at least two things you won't eat because they're nutritionally unsound?
48 Feel that your diet will help you live a longer life?

Here is some space in which you can generate additional activities . . . your own curriculum-development practicum. You can do it!

Moral dilemmas

What would you do if:

1 Your doctor told you to cut out all ice cream?
2 Your doctor told you to cut out all chocolate?
3 A friend offered to trade you a cupcake for your carrots?
4 You were on a diet and were served a rich dessert when having dinner with friends?
5 One of your friends ate only TV dinners?
6 You forbade your children to have soft drinks, and you discovered they were drinking them while at friends' houses?
7 The person at your house who cooks always overcooks the vegetables?
8 You wanted to make Thanksgiving more than a time to "stuff your mouth"?
9 You felt deceived by TV commercials about the nutritional content of certain foods?
10 You were a guest at someone's home and didn't like the taste of the main dish?
11 You were at a restaurant, asked for your meat rare, and found it to be well-done?
12 You caught someone on a diet sneaking a piece of pie?
13 Someone you love is overeating?
14 You saw a parent promising his or her child a piece of candy if the child were good?
15 You saw someone drinking four cups of coffee each morning?
16 You noticed that one of your classmates never had a dessert packed?
17 One of your friends who has acne always ordered French fries?
18 Your father is putting on weight and keeps insisting on seconds on potatoes?
19 You wanted to get your family to eat less—without nagging them?
20 A person says he or she is on a diet, and then comes off it in your presence?

Here is some space in which you can generate additional activities . . . your own curriculum-development practicum. You can do it!

Spread of opinion

1 Junkin' Jack ————————————————————— Pure Paul

Jack's diet consists solely of junk foods—he even goes so far as to make sure there is no nutrition in any of the foods he purchases. Paul also looks at the labels of the food he purchases—and calculates to the fourth decimal point the percentage of nutrients. Paul is a known health gnat—he's always bugging people about getting enough nutrition.

2 Low-cost Carla ————————————————————— Expensive Edna

When shopping, Carla will search high and low . . . mostly low . . . for the cheapest brands. She doesn't loaf around even when it involves buying discount bread that is a week old. On the other hand, Edna feels that the more expensive a brand is, the better it is. She avoids sales at all costs, figuring that there must be something wrong with the food if it doesn't cost a lot.

3 Dieting Dierdre ————————————————————— Sneaking Stan

Dierdre is a real diet-hard. When she decides to go on a diet, no temptation in the world can pull her off it. Stan, on the other hand, will go on a diet just so he can take up the challenge of finding creative ways to break it.

4 Nibbling Nelly ————————————————————— Fourths Fran

Nelly is a person who always seems to eat around her food. She takes very small portions and always seems to leave most of her food on the plate. Fran is unabashed about asking for seconds, thirds, fourths, and is known as the human dishwasher; her plate is always wiped clean.

Here is some space in which you can generate additional activities . . . your own curriculum-development practicum. You can do it!

Inventory

1. *Foods that you enjoy snacking on*

    A You usually eat it alone.
    P You usually eat it with another person(s) present.
    T You often eat it while watching TV.
    F It's fattening.
    C You have considered giving it up.
    A You have seen it advertised on TV.

2. *Refrigerator survey—what's in yours?*

    P Your parents bought the item.
    $ One of the more expensive brands.
    * Your five favorite foods in the refrigerator.
    S You like to pack your lunch for school.
    + A food you have only on special occasions.
    N A food you consider to be nutritious.

3. *The ways you are nourished*

    F Through food.
    A Through physical affection, touching.
    C Through compliments.
    P Your parents nourish you in this way.
    Y You nourish others in this way.
    + You nourish yourself in this way.

4. *An ideal meal*

    M Would be on your mother's list.
    F Would be on your father's list.
    X Would not have been on your list five years ago.
    I Will be on your list for your entire life.
    Y Yummy, it tastes good!
    H Healthful food.

Here is some space in which you can generate additional activities . . . your own currriculum-development practicum. You can do it!

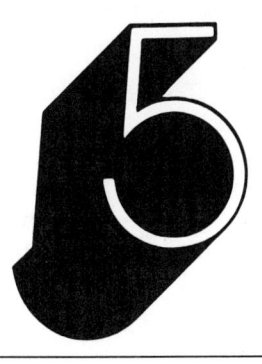

5
WRITING ACTIVITIES

In the following pages, you will find additional strategies in the areas of human sexuality and family life; drugs; and nutrition.

These strategies differ from those we have just presented in that, in each case, these strategies are set up in such a way that they can be handed out to the student rather than presented verbally.

Thus, these represent examples of how you may be able to allow students to work on their own, either in small groups at school, or at home. We call these *writing* strategies because they specifically channel students into putting pen to paper.

An important aspect of these is your stress to the students that you will not be correcting grammar, spelling, and punctuation in the material they present.

THE PERSONAL DIARY

Asking students to keep a personal diary or journal provides an excellent writing strategy. This follows up on the ideas of Maslow, who found that clues to personal characteristics come from biographical material.

Thus, it could be extremely meaningful to your students if you were to encourage them to keep a personal diary or journal of their thoughts, feelings in relation to the class, exercises, and relationships outside class.

Students can then be asked to reread their journal at some point, as though they had found it on a street. They can write a brief description of the individual about whom they have just read, and make comments and observations about this person. Particularly, have your students look at their strengths, successes, and how they can build on these in terms of their own lives.

STRATEGIES IN HUMAN SEXUALITY

Is this me?

Consider each description carefully and ask yourself the question, "Is this me?" On the continuum below, place the number for each description in that position that best applies to you.

Description

1 Feel positive about myself.
2 Like all people.
3 Very critical of other people.
4 Very critical of myself.
5 Am spontaneous.
6 Am a follower.
7 Am a leader.
8 Good son (or daughter).
9 Full of energy.
10 Hard-working.
11 Can be trusted.
12 Ready to help.

True of me   Could be   Not me at all

1   Could you write one "I learned . . ." statement here?

Professional roles

Below are listed various career opportunities. Your task is to rate each career as to how favorable or unfavorable you feel about it as a career for you. (This rating does not apply to your ability to function in this career, but is used only to get in touch with how the career appeals to you.) Use the following rating scale:

1   *Would like to pursue.*
2   *Would consider.*
3   *Uncertain.*
4   *Doubt that I would consider.*
5   *Would never consider.*

89 WRITING ACTIVITIES Chapter 5

CAREER	RATING	CAREER	RATING
nurse	_____	bank teller	_____
elementary-school teacher	_____	truck driver	_____
hairdresser	_____	disc jockey	_____
plumber	_____	doctor	_____
secretary	_____	dentist	_____
jockey	_____	dental hygienist	_____
cashier	_____	writer	_____
college professor	_____	airplane pilot	_____
telephone operator	_____	veterinarian	_____
bartender	_____	lawyer	_____
operator of day care center	_____	taxi driver	_____
electrician	_____	salesclerk	_____

1 *Look over your list. Do you see a pattern in your answers which might suggest a "sexist" attitude toward career choices? Explain:*

2 *See if you can list five things that you can do that the opposite sex cannot do:*

Sexual freedom

Theoretically this is a free country, but sometimes we are less free than at other times.

Directions:

Think of two times or places when or where you feel most sexually free, and two situations where you do not feel sexually free. Describe them in the spaces provided. For each example, explain whether it refers to freedom *from* something or someone, or freedom *to* do something.

1 *Two times or places when or where I feel most sexually free:*

2 *Two times or places when or where I do not feel sexually free:*

3 *Can you write one "I learned" (or "I re-learned") statement below?*

Men and women　Below are a number of statements concerning male/female roles. See if you can respond to them as thoroughly as possible.

1 *Steve and Barbara were married while graduate students at State University. Both received their Ph.D.'s at the same time. Steve was offered a very good job in San Francisco. Barbara was offered a top job in her field in Houston, Texas. What do you feel they should do?*

2 *What are your feelings concerning this article from "Dear Abby"?*

Dear Abby: Why do mothers teach their daughters that when a boy brings them home from a date they should "thank" him for the lovely evening? After all it's the man who does the asking, and if the lady *grants* him the date, then *he* should thank her for the lovely evening.

3 *The statement, "I do it for twenty bucks, she does it for a steak dinner, what's the difference?" was recently made by a prostitute speaking on television. What are your feelings about this statement?*

4 *See if you can list five things that you can do that the opposite sex cannot.*

Fantasies about marriage　　Many of us have all kinds of fantasies concerning marriage and the roles that people have in marriage. Whether you are married or do not plan to get married at this time (if at all), see if you can write out one fantasy (an ideal or wish) that you have about marriage, in the brief space provided. Attempt to focus on something to which you have given some thought.

91 WRITING ACTIVITIES   Chapter 5

Below are listed various roles in marriage. See if you can rate them in terms of how they relate to your expectations about marriage and the roles you see yourself playing. Use the following rating scale:

1   See myself in this role.
2   I may consider this role.
3   Uncertain at this time.
4   I doubt that I would consider this role.
5   I would never consider this role.

Rating   Role

____ The major breadwinner in the family.

____ Housekeeper and cook.

____ Cook part of the time.

____ Clean the house part of the time.

____ Stay home and take care of the children.

____ Take care of the money.

____ See to the upkeep of the car.

____ Do the wash.

____ Take care of the grocery shopping.

____ Work part-time at a job and part-time in the home.

____ Be the boss in the family.

____ Take care of the kids while my spouse goes on a trip.

____ Pay the bills.

Feelings about my body

Various parts of (or conditions of) your body are listed below. See if you can rate each part, using the following rating scale:

1   Am really happy with it.
2   Am satisfied with it.
3   No feelings either way.
4   Don't like but can tolerate it.
5   Am unhappy with it and would like to change it.

____ face   ____ neck

____ complexion   ____ chest

____ hair   ____ arms

____ nose   ____ hands

____ eyes   ____ waist

___ butt   ___ body build

___ hips   ___ thighs

___ genitals   ___ body hair

___ knees   ___ stomach

___ legs   ___ posture

___ feet   ___ back

___ weight   ___ ankles

___ height   ___ overall body

1 *Choose one part of your body that you really like and take a minute to discuss briefly what it is that you really like about that part of your body.*

2 *Can you write one "I learned . . ." statement here?*

I agree about marriage

Look over the statements below. Circle only those you can most agree with.

Marriages are made in heaven.

Love is all that is necessary for a good marriage.

Marriage is for the birds.

You can love two people at the same time.

Sex is the most important single factor in marriage.

Sex outside of marriage is wrong.

A woman's place is in the home.

The male is the head of the family.

A marriage without children is only half a family.

Two people must have the same interests in order to stay together.

Love changes with age.

Two people can marry and yet not love one another.

Adultery is always wrong.

Jealousy can be a very positive emotion.

93 WRITING ACTIVITIES Chapter 5

Varieties in sexual intercourse are important in marriage.

The open-ended marriage is a form of adultery.

Love and sex are different.

Sexuality and sensuality are the same.

1 *Look over your circles. Are the circled statements compatible with each other?*

2 *Go over your list with someone else in your class, or have your date/mate also go through the list and then compare answers.*

Forced choice See if you can make a forced choice by marking one of three decisions based on the following stories:

	WON'T ACCEPT	UNSURE	ACCEPT
1. Someone you find yourself falling in love with tells you he/she is having a relationship with someone else but still loves you.	___	___	___
2. Your spouse says that he/she would like to try living in a commune for a while.	___	___	___
3. Your spouse of five years says that love has never existed but he/she still wants to keep the marriage going.	___	___	___
4. Your spouse suggests to you that he/she would like to have a sexual relationship with someone else.	___	___	___
5. You find out that the person you are about to marry is bisexual.	___	___	___
6. Your spouse suggests adopting a young child of another race.	___	___	___
7. Your spouse would rather adopt children than have children through pregnancy.	___	___	___

Your choice Consider these questions and reflect:

1 *Given the opportunity to have a child through selective breeding (i.e. in a test tube) with a guarantee of no defects, would you still want to have your baby in the traditional fashion—with no guarantee?*

2   *Would you like the opportunity to determine the sex, hair, eye color, and other physical attributes of your child?*
3   *Can you see the concept of positive eugenics as the answer to the improvement of the human species?*
4   *Should medical authorities have the final say as to who, based on genetic favorability-unfavorability, should have and not have children?*

Sexual ads

There are various ways of finding a sex partner. Some place "personal" want ads in newspapers, some advertise through friends, some "advertise" through the use of clothing.

Directions:

Quickly read over the "personals" below and ask yourself the question: "Which one most intrigues me, and to which might I respond?"

Intelligent sensitive male, age 34, desires pretty, shapely female, 18-35 who is warm, affectionate and understanding. I am 5'8", medium build, average looking, talented, compassionate & understanding, with a sense of humor. I like music, cultural activities & sports. If you desire a sincere, honest, romantic relationship and companionship & would enjoy being needed & appreciated, then please write to: I.S., P.O. Box 000, New York, N.Y. (photo optional).	Very beautiful girl under 26 years desired for marriage to 37 year, 6' tall slender, considerate, warm professional. Write: L. Hogan, 0000 Crescent St., Queens, L.I.C., N.Y.	Generous Grad. student; 27, 6'2", 175, Cauc., Shy, Moustached. Seeks female (only) sexual partners for casual relationships. Age, Race no barrier. 609 - 000-0000. Collect 10-11:30 p.m.	Young male, (23), good-looking, medium build, 5'10", interested in music, literature, politics, etc., desires to share life in serious, hopefully long-term relationship with same. Must be good-looking, intelligent, unaffected, under 24 yrs. No brutes, no creeps, no psychos. Write, give background ad lib., enclose photos (portrait) — Box 000, Cathedral Station, N.Y., N.Y. 10025. If interested will reciprocate promptly and, if mutually satisfactory, will arrange meeting. Absolute discretion assured.
	Male 29 desires to meet mature women, for mutual desirable sex relations. Also has friend if you have one. Reply to: Box 0000 GPO NYC, N.Y. 10001	Tall, handsome professional man seeks uninhibited female. G.P.O. Box 0000, Brooklyn, N.Y.	
Tall, handsome young male artist (32, 6'3", 185lbs.), needs lovely young nympho type girl friend for lunches and daytime or twilight togetherness. Call 000-0000, days.	Young man in 20's desires a sincere relationship and offers a home (the upper east side) to a female who enjoys taking care of a house and a man (not financially). Please write to: Mr. Lemis, P.O. Box 00, Prince St. Sta. NY, NY 10012.	TO THE GAL WHO LEADS A DOUBLE LIFE (OR WOULD LIKE TO): Considerate, good-looking businessman (35) with luxury apartment and cultured tastes (music, theater, art, travel, sports cars), solid citizen by day, unmasks after dark. Seeks slim, lovely, intelligent gal companion or roommate. Phone Mr. Carr during office hours. 000-0000	Love, love, love...if you need it — we're sexperts. Two guys with groovy ideas for fun and pleasure Call Billy 000-0000 or Allen 000-0000 evenings.
Man, late 20's, seeks FEMALE partner, for indoor nudist gatherings. Only twenty minutes from NYC. Female callers only. Call 201 - 000-0000 from 6-9 p.m. only.	Attractive professional man, 20's seeks friendly, unspoiled, uninhibited female, to lead to meaningful relationship. Write: Box 000, Bronx 10453.	Two young, handsome men await nympho type girls, preferably women, seeking to have sexual relationship. Please write, accompanied by photo (intriguing) if possible. No homos. 00 Carle Rd., Westbury, L.I.	Cameraman in Boston on feature film offers sweet, young, pretty swinger(s) chance of a lifetime to meet actors, film-makers and technicians from N.Y. and Hollywood. Call Ross (617) 000-0000 or send photo, 000 Boylston St.. No wierdos or prudes, please.
ORAL LOVE — Good looking magazine editor in mid-twenties desires FEMALE partner (18-30) for wild and discreet love making sessions. I can and will do anything with the right girl. Call John Buhle 000-0000, leave name and number. NO fags, please.	Imaginative young male disciplinarian desires relationship with obedient, receptive young female in Boston Area. Write "DM" c/o P.O. Box 00, Newton Center, Mass. 02159	Young man 32, own Manhattan apartment would like to meet girl 20-30 who desires mature companionship. Call Michael, 000-0000 late in evenings.	Our group, swinging in the NYC, NJ and Philadelphia areas, seeks discreet, attractive girls, guys and couples interested in the Libidinal laws of nature. A description of yourself & photo appreciated. Write: P.O. Box 00 Winslow Post Office, NJ 08095
Tall, attractive, mature Spanish artist, 34 with apartment in West Village looking for quiet attractive female to share love, art and bed games. 8 a.m. or after 10 p.m. 000-0000.	WANTED: Interesting, sexy, young girl for afternoon or evening dates with man, 30, tall, intelligent, generous, village apartment. PO Box 000, Cooper Station, NY. 10003	Cultured, successful gentleman interested in the arts - theatre, ballet, all music, etc. Would like to meet an intelligent, attractive gal to enjoy same. Be my guest, winter vacation in the islands and late spring, summer in Europe. May consider financial help for talented, creative girl. Have beautiful midtown pad which you may share. Phone anytime (212) 000-0000 and let's wine and dine.	Magic math: one times one times sixty-nine equals Zowie. Free tuition for succulent goddess. Send nude Polaroid and phone to Studio One, 000 West 58 St., New York 10019, pronto.
YOU'RE SENSITIVE, a grown-up girl who loves conversation, delights in the hay? Share tall, traveled writer's warmth, bread . . . pad? Jay Robideaux, (NYC) 000-0000 (messages).	Professional man, 29 — wanted young, warm, uninhibited, intelligent WOMAN 18-35, to share bright apt. on a mutually satisfying basis. No Homo's Call Bob after 6: Phone 000-0000 or Write: Bob - apt. 4, 0000 74th St., 11373 N.Y.		Good looking business executive White, 33, 6'2", well endowed seeks attractive girls or couples for intimate get-togethers. NY - NJ area. I own color polaroid if interested. Photo, phone a must. Write: W. Davis, P.O. Box 000, Ansonia Sta. NYC 10023
30 year old very handsome executive desires to learn about cunnilingus. Write Stuart Rivers c/o Craft Service, W. 74th St. NYC.	Attractive, female art teacher, young, recently divorced, seeks swinging boy and girl friends for physical and emotional fun. Will call or Write. Box 00 Oakland Gardens, Flushing, NY	Quietness of the mind can be found!! Even in the void of the learning room of machines . . . ZOD	

WRITING ACTIVITIES   Chapter 5

1 *To which of these ads would you consider responding?*

Directions:

Write a "personal" ad of your own below. You have from 25 to 30 words to write it in so be specific.

STRATEGIES IN DRUG EDUCATION

Drugs and me

On the left side of the line make a list of all the drugs that you can think of. Don't forget to include such "soft" and "hard" drugs as alcohol, tobacco, marijuana, heroin, etc. When you are done, move on to the next page.

Drug List | Code

After you have made your list you may wish to share it with the group. You may have some drugs listed that they don't and that they can add. Go back over your list and on the right side of your paper add the code system to your list:

D *All those drugs you feel are dangerous to the user in some way.*
HU *Those drugs you have used, but have since stopped using.*
SU *Those drugs you are still using.*
*Going back over the list of drugs you are now using and adding the approximate number of times you have used that drug in the last month.*
? *Those drugs you are curious about using and may try, given the right opportunity.*
P *Those drugs that have been used in your presence but which you have not used yourself.*
I *Those drugs you feel should be illegal.*

Directions:

Below are a number of statements about drugs. Respond to each statement by *circling* the response that best describes how you feel:

SA *Strongly agree.*
A *Agree.*
N *Neutral.*
D *Disagree.*
SD *Strongly disagree.*

1	I have a tendency to drink too much.	SA A N D SD
2	I have a tendency to drink just because my friends drink.	SA A N D SD
3	I feel a lot better about myself when I am not using drugs.	SA A N D SD
4	I like to get drunk when I drink.	SA A N D SD
5	I never worry about my drug use, even though I do a lot of drugs.	SA A N D SD
6	I always feel that I can drive a car even though I have had a lot to drink.	SA A N D SD
7	I use drugs just to be one of the gang.	SA A N D SD
8	I like to get drunk at parties.	SA A N D SD
9	I prefer to do a number of different drugs at the same time, like drinking and smoking pot.	SA A N D SD
10	I like to drink when I am alone.	SA A N D SD
11	I am concerned about my drug use.	SA A N D SD
12	I would like to talk with someone about my drug use.	SA A N D SD

1 *Can you write one "I learned . . ." statement here?*

What's your response?

Given the below situations what would you do?

	YES	NO
1. Do you automatically take "a few" aspirin each time you have a pain or headache?	___	___
2. When you have a cold, do you automatically go to the drugstore for a new supply of cold pills?	___	___
3. Do you (or would you) automatically take, without question, any drugs prescribed by your doctor?	___	___
4. Do you ever think about the adverse effects that certain "safe" drugs such as aspirin can have on you?	___	___
5. Do you tend to accept most commercial statements that are made through ads and TV concerning drugs?	___	___
6. Have you ever considered the possibilities of a drug-free state of mind and body; that is, giving up all drugs such as aspirin, coffee, cold pills, alcohol, and so on?	___	___

Consider your responses to these questions. Then make some observations about your answers to these questions:

1 *What do you consider "safe" and "unsafe" drugs?*

2 *Can you suggest one alternative to the use of such drugs as aspirin?*

3 *What would you suggest as an alternative model to drug use?*

STRATEGIES IN NUTRITION EDUCATION

Favorite foods First, go over the lists and circle those foods you have eaten in the past week. Next, go over the lists again and cross out all those foods you rarely, if ever, eat.

VEGETABLES	MEATS	FRUITS	DAIRY
asparagus	bacon	apples	butter
beans	chicken	bananas	cheese
beets	frankfurters	berries	cream
cabbage	fish	grapefruit	eggs
carrots	ham	grapes	ice cream
cauliflower	hamburger	lemons	margarine
celery	lamb chops	melon	milk
corn	pork chops	oranges	Other:
cucumbers	roast beef	peaches	_____
lettuce	salami	pears	_____
mushrooms	steak	Other:	_____
onions	sausage	_____	BAKERY
peas	turkey	_____	bread
potatoes	Other:	_____	cake
spinach	_____		cookies
squash	_____		crackers
tomatoes	_____		muffins
turnips			pie
Other:			rolls
_____			Other:
_____			_____
_____			_____

Compare your responses to "Favorite Foods" with a partner:

1 *List the responses that are similar.*

WRITING ACTIVITIES Chapter 5

2 *Were there choices that were quite different? If so, list these.*

3 *What reasons can you offer that might account for the differences between the two appraisals?*

4 *Which list do you feel makes more sense nutritionally? Why?*

I would rather

Look at the "I would rather" statements below and circle in each column the one that most applies to you. If neither applies, then circle "neither."

I WOULD RATHER

eat	than	sleep	neither
eat	than	drink	neither
eat eggs	than	eat meat	neither
eat vegetables	than	eat meat	neither
eat meat	than	eat fish	neither
drink soda	than	drink milk	neither
drink tea	than	drink coffee	neither
spend money on food	than	spend money on books	neither
eat a lot	than	eat a little	neither
eat a lot at one time	than	eat a little at one time	neither
study	than	eat	neither
eat what I like	than	eat what might be healthful	neither
eat and the hell with cholesterol	than	be very concerned with cholesterol	neither
drink nonfat milk	than	whole milk	neither

1 *Can you write one "I learned . . ." statement below?*

6

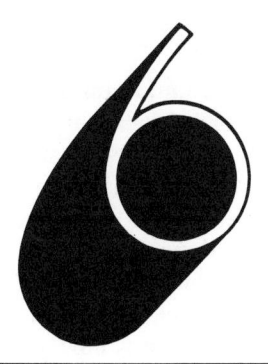

WORKING THROUGH AN EXERCISE

One Particularly Effective Seating Arrangement

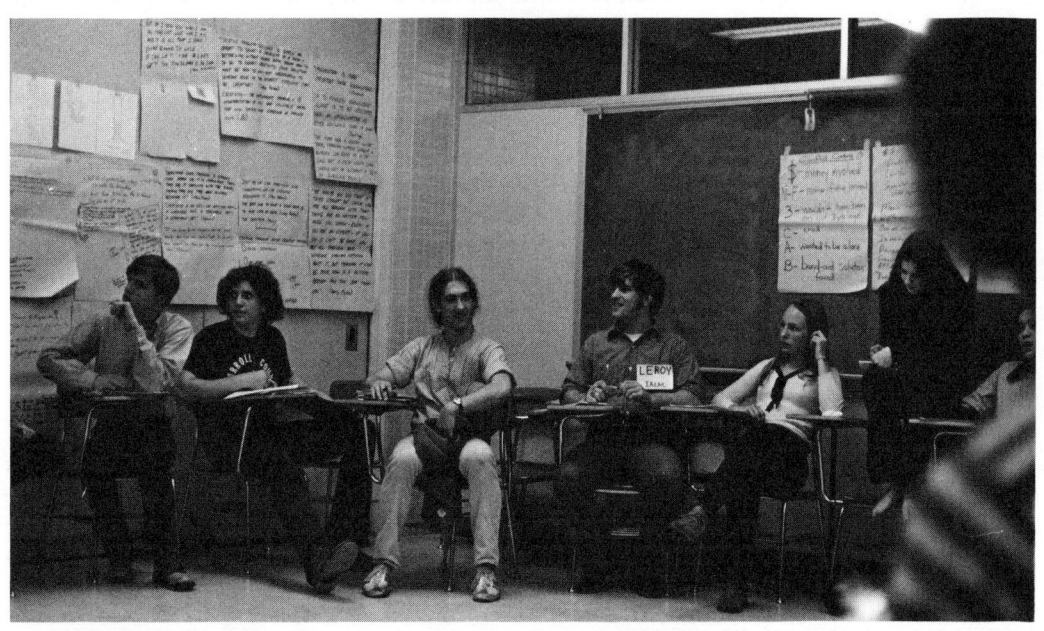

A seating arrangement in which students are allowed to sit (either in chairs or on the floor) in a circle has been found by the authors to be extremely effective. Most important is that the teacher become part of that circle.

Processing an exercise is the most important and valuable aspect of the values-clarification approach, for it is here that students begin to gain greater insights into their own values. It is here that they often begin to ask such questions or make such statements as: "Do I really feel this way?" "Is what I am saying consistent with what I am doing?" "Do I feel good about what I have said or done?" "I'm OK after all!" "Boy—did I learn something new about myself today!"

Statements such as these are often felt and overheard when one has gone through an experience or exercise and is now in the processing stage of sharing feelings.

STEPPING BACK FOR A MINUTE

Before we get into processing, it may be a good idea if we cover some of the important first things a teacher should consider before working with a particular value exercise.

First

The teacher should spend some time planning for work with a particular value exercise. Certainly here also the teacher should give some consideration to which strategy or combination of strategies she/he wishes to work with. This should, to a great degree, depend on such things as:

a subject matter being covered;
b specific issues the students are anxious to work on;
c areas the teacher feels are important and need to be clarified; and
d time allocation—do you, and can you, have five minutes, 30 minutes, an hour, half a day? You should set a time limit AND STICK TO IT.

Second

Is the exercise you choose to use the right one for the situation? That is, are the students ready? Can they handle the exercise? Is the atmosphere in the classroom such that you can expect a high degree of support and honesty? These and other questions should be answered, especially before you venture into working with "high-risk" exercises. And any high-risk exercise requires a great degree of *trust* in the classroom.

Third

After you have decided on what exercise you would like to use, you should then have some idea of the materials (if any) you will need to work with. Questions you might consider here are:

a   can I use the room that I am now in as it is or will I have to rearrange chairs and other items to some degree?
b   is there a need for handouts, or can students supply all needs for the activity? and,
c   does the activity or exercise require students to be active—and, if so, all the students or just some?

Fourth

Observation is an important aspect of working with any exercise that requires students to get in touch with their personal feelings and values. The teacher should accept a certain degree of responsibility for seeing to it that students feel that they may share, do not put each other down, and do not use "killer statements." It goes without saying that the role of the teacher-facilitator is that of guiding the process in such a way that the environment (the classroom) provides a setting in which students do not feel threatened or put down when sharing (or attempting to share) their feelings.

The teacher should be constantly on the alert to stay in touch with students in terms of where they are and what they are feeling. In short, the teacher should have a "feel" for what is going on in the classroom.

The teacher should also be aware of those students who do not wish to share and should see to it thay they are *not* forced to do so by other students.

SOME KILLER STATEMENTS

asinine	it will never work
bad idea	nonsense
can't do it	not feasible
contrary to my thinking	nutty
cornball	loony
crackpot idea	moronic
crappy	out of the question
crazy	pathetic
crummy	ridiculous
doesn't make sense	stupid
doesn't sound good	thumbs down
don't believe it	too extreme
dopey	too screwy
dumb idea	unacceptable
get serious	unimaginative
have you flipped?	unrealistic
idiotic	useless
I disagree	weird
imbecilic	worthless
insane	you're crazy
it's stupid	you're nuts
it stinks	you've got to be kidding

Every Child A "Winner"

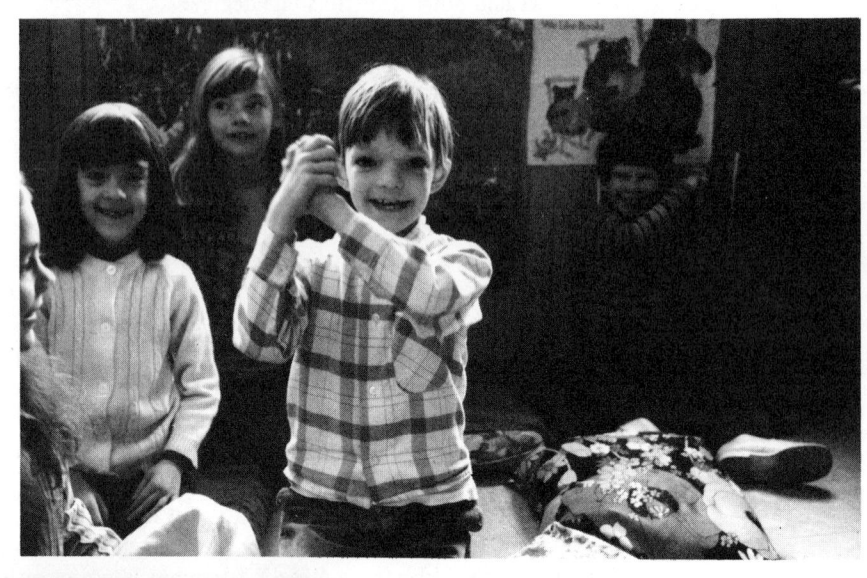

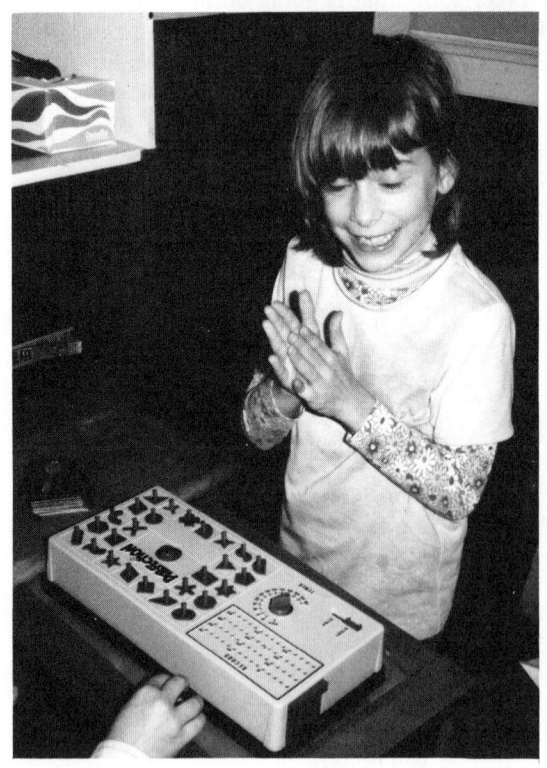

The best type of self-concept building there is.

Fifth

Finally, after the allocated amount of time has been used in going through an exercise, you may now want time to do some processing. Some of the important stages in processing include:

a   Allowing time for students to review their feelings and behavior as they were working through the activity or exercise. Here you may wish to ask them such clarifying questions as: "How did you feel as you worked on [or through] the exercise?" "Did you consistently change your mind?" "Did you learn anything new about yourself as you worked through the activity?" "Did you recognize any differences between others and yourself?" "Are your responses consistent with your behavior?"

b   At the end of the exercise or activity you may wish to have students share a "one word" feeling. Go around the room and have them share aloud. Try to keep each one to an expression or feeling word.

c   Other questions you may wish to consider asking students, either in small support groups or in a large group, include: "Did you find yourself being 'active' or 'passive', or a 'leader' or 'follower' during the exercise?" "Could you share one 'I learned . . .' statement?" "Can you identify any patterns that occurred in how you felt, behaved, or responded"? "If you could repeat the exercise is there anything you would do differently?" "Did you respond any differently from the way you usually do?"

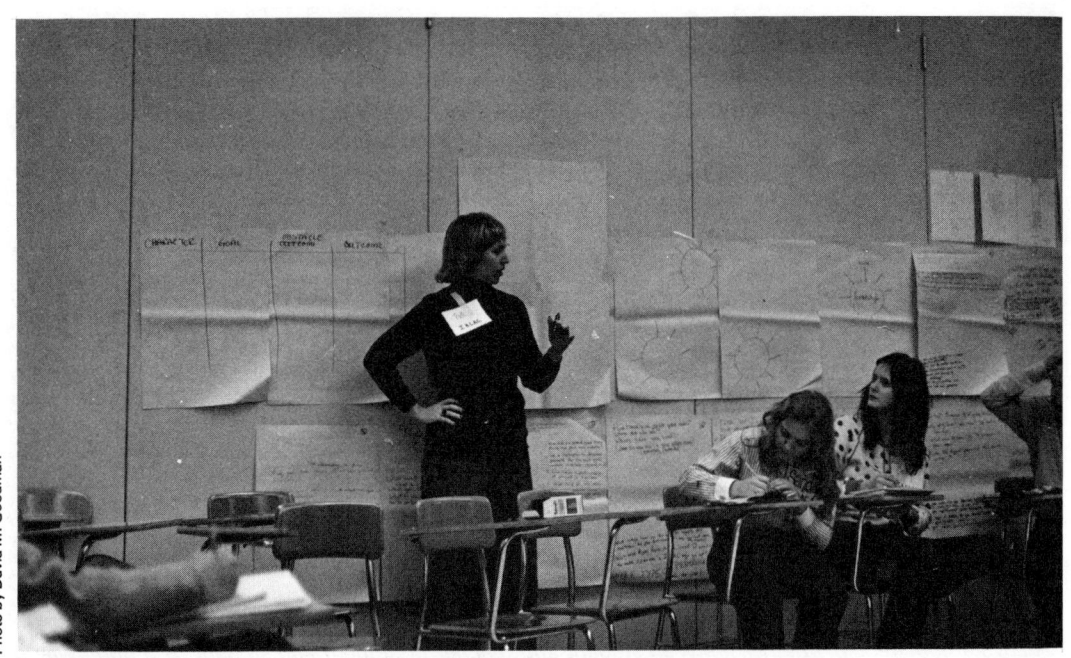

Dealing with "unfinished business" is an extremely important aspect of the teaching-learning process. This is especially true when students have been dealing with some highly emotional material such as human sexuality.

106 HEALTH EDUCATION: THE SEARCH FOR VALUES

Finally

At the end of an activity or exercise you should *always* try to deal with any unfinished business that might interfere with the functioning of the class. This process might include one or more people.

Sometimes simply asking the question: "Is there any unfinished business that someone has and would like to share?" or "Is there something someone would like to say?" or "I sense there is some unfinished business!" is helpful. Always deal with such unfinished business if you sense that it does exist. But don't push. If a student who you sense is dealing with certain feelings does not want to share, that's all right too. You may want to suggest a private conference. Finally, remember that the unfinished business may be in you.

To bring closure to the group, you may want to gather the whole group together (if they are in their support groups) for one or two minutes of group sharing. Here too, you may be able to share certain feelings of your own as a way of opening up the group.

You may also at this point want to do some group validating —that is, sharing your feelings about the class and certain students in the class by saying such things as: "I want to thank Bill for sharing what he did!" "Sue for being so open and honest!" "Judy for going out of her way to help Jim!"

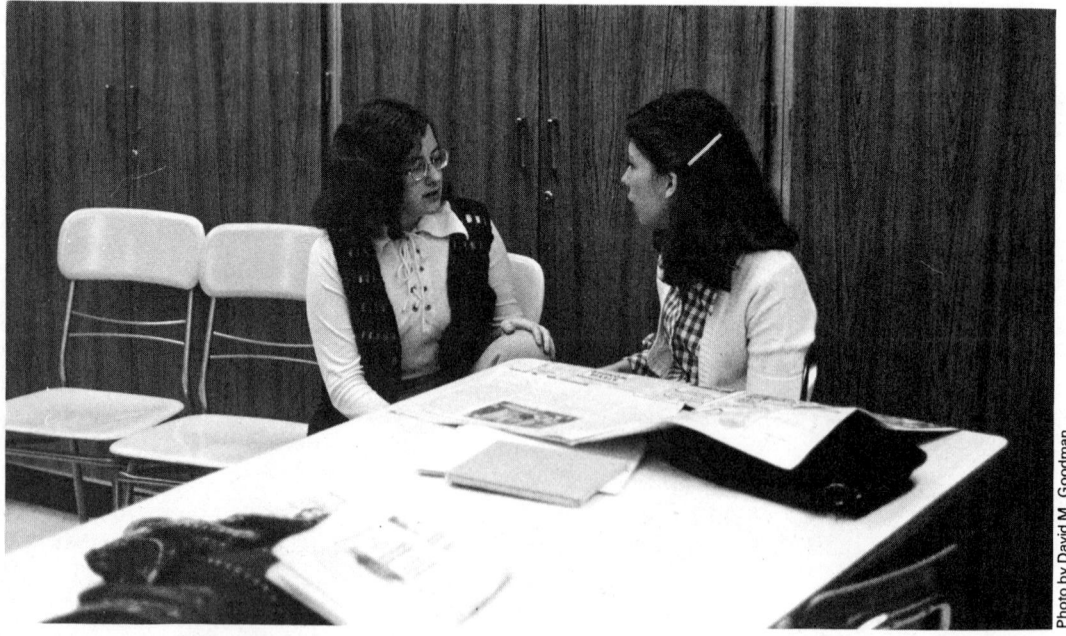

A private conference, whether between student and teacher or student and student, is a good way of dealing with any unfinished business of the day.

1

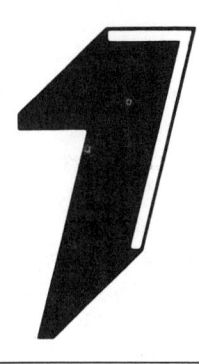

PROCESSING

What we are going to do here is to take you through two exercises. This, we hope, will give you some feeling for working with values strategies.

It should be pointed out that these activities are designed primarily to involve the students' personal feelings and experiences. It is, therefore, important that you create a supportive, nonjudgmental classroom environment. Some students will be reluctant to look at themselves, much less reveal themselves to others. Students will be open about themselves only to the degree that an atmosphere of safety and trust is created.

Stress should be put on the idea that these exercises are not designed to uncover any serious emotional problems. As stated earlier, if a student finds an activity threatening, or is reluctant to join with the class or group in any discussion, you should respect the student's attitude. Here too, private conference outside of the class may help the student overcome any personal concerns.

Try to help the class develop a healthy respect for differences of opinion. Make it clear that the individuality of each student should be highly valued. In group discussions, encourage the full participation of each and every student, but also make certain that students know they have a right to "pass." Remember that effective group techniques (e.g. positive focus, trust) may be introduced to insure maximum individual participation and learning.

Overall, the way in which you use a method or exercise is probably far more important than which method or exercise you use.[1] What is even more important is that you set an atmosphere that will give students confidence that their personal feelings and values, no matter how they differ from others (and yours), are legitimate and respected by you and others. Encourage them continually to express their feelings and values. This can be done in class discussions, small-group work (in support groups), individual one-to-one conferences, and projects (such as in a personal diary). Of course, these methods and techniques in no way guarantee openness and trust. If a teacher attempts to manipulate small groups or discussions, or if a teacher is "right-answer" oriented, students will be intimidated regardless of the method being used.

EXERCISE: NAME TAGS

This activity is frequently used as an "icebreaker" or first-day activity in small or large groups. It helps students get acquainted quickly and easily and also offers a way of learning first names. At a deeper level, however, it may also help students to increase their awareness of each other's uniqueness as a person, with different ideas and opinions.

Working through

Provide each student with a large name tag. Self-adhesive labels, if large, work well, as do large index cards or colored paper with a strong pin. Ask each person to write his or her first name in the middle of the tag, using a large felt-tip marker. Have them leave space around the outside for some additional information.

Describe the activity to the class as a get-acquainted exercise in which members will meet their fellow classmates and find out some things that they value. You might explain that in their work this year, it will be important that they know and trust each other. Many of the activities that will follow in class will depend upon their being able to share their feelings and experiences.

Choose four (or more if you desire) items from the list below and read them to the class. Each student is to record his/her responses to each item, writing it with pen or pencil in the section of the card that you have indicated. Example:

"In the upper right-hand corner of your card write down the name of an animal that you feel best represents your feelings!"

[1] See Joel Goodman and Marie Hartwell Walker's "Affective Ed—A Means, Not an End," *Learning,* January 1976, p. 52.

"IALAC"

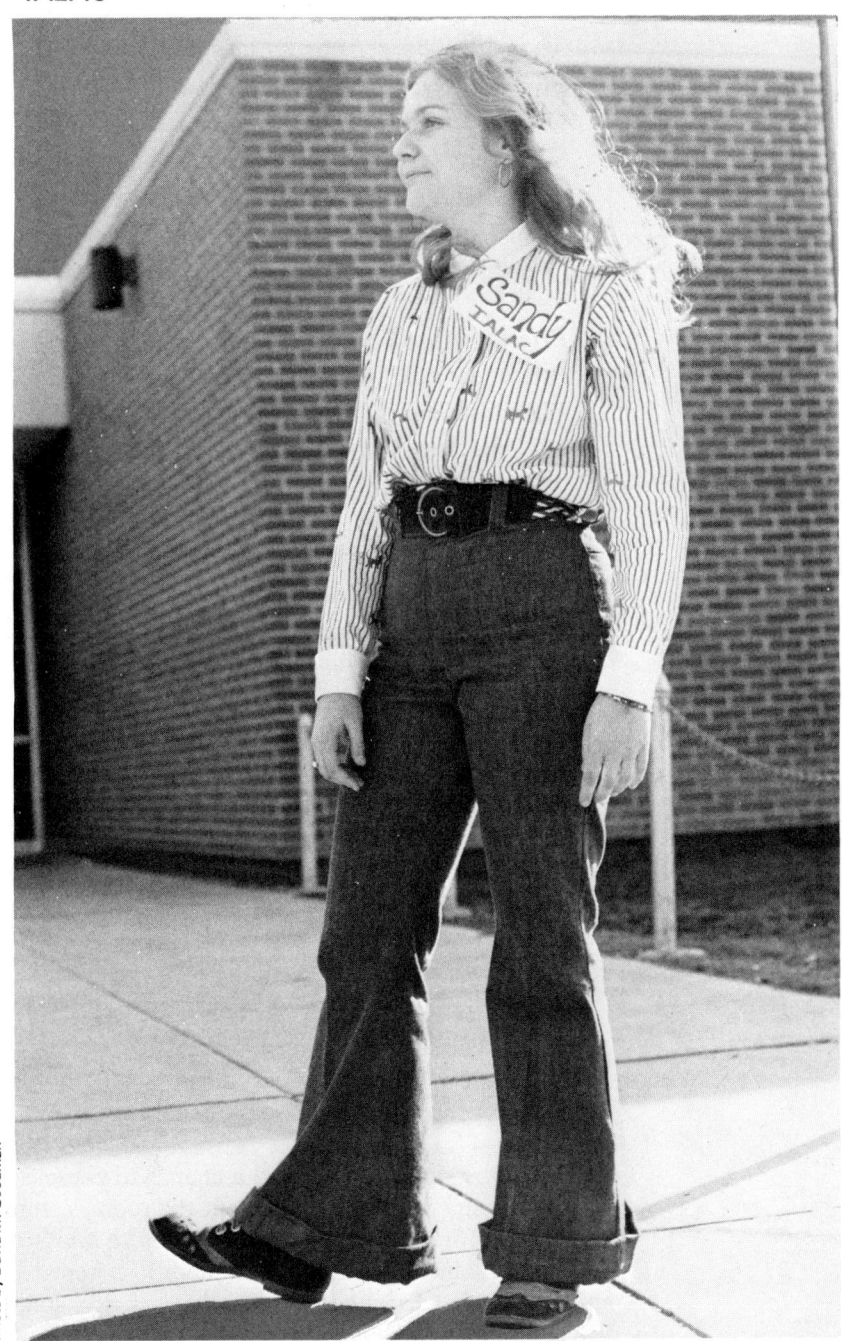

The allegory on the classical put-down: "I Am Loveable And Capable", from a story made popular by Sidney B. Simon.

Additional items that you may want to consider include:

The name of a person you most admire.
Five things you like about yourself.
One aspect of your physical self that you like the most.
Something you have been wanting to say for a long time.
How would you describe yourself in three words?
Something you could teach the rest of the class.
The name you would call yourself if you could have chosen your name.
Five adjectives beginning with the words "I am someone who . . ."
Briefly describe your personal Utopia.
The most important object in your life.
Five things that would describe you that you would put in a time capsule.
Five objectives you have for your life.
Write a brief obituary of yourself.
Three things that make you happy.
Three things you do well.
What are your hobbies?
What is your favorite movie? Song? Book?
What games did you play when you were young?
Where was your favorite hiding place?
What did you want to be when you were very young?
What things were you not allowed to do when you were young?
List any family traditions.
Can you list one favorite toy you had as a child?
Five significant things in your wallet or pocketbook.
Three significant people in your life—both past as well as present.
The name of your old girl friend/boy friend.
The name of a book that you have read more than once.
The first three things you did this morning.

When the students have had a chance to complete their personal card, encourage them to move about the room, comparing their responses. Moving freely from one person to another helps classmates become acquainted with each other and, it is hoped, more comfortable with each other. During this icebreaker activity, students will discover differences in individuals; the realization of this is a first step toward trust and acceptance.

A Group-sharing Session.

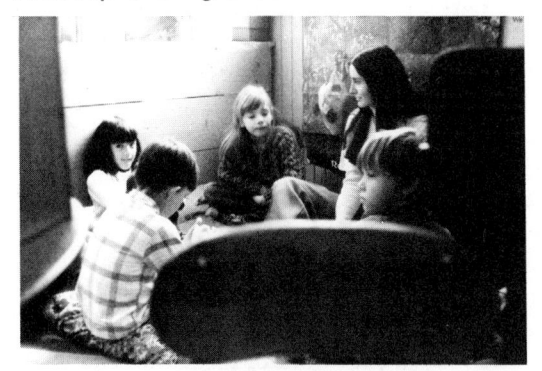

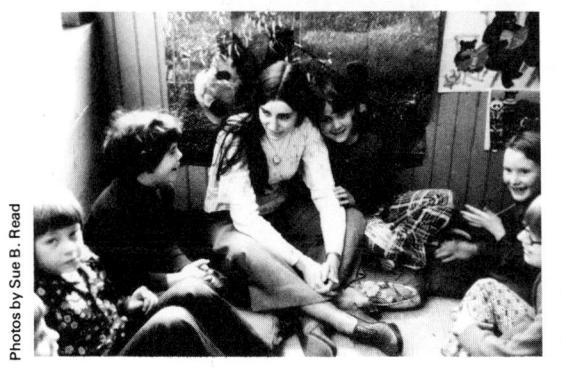

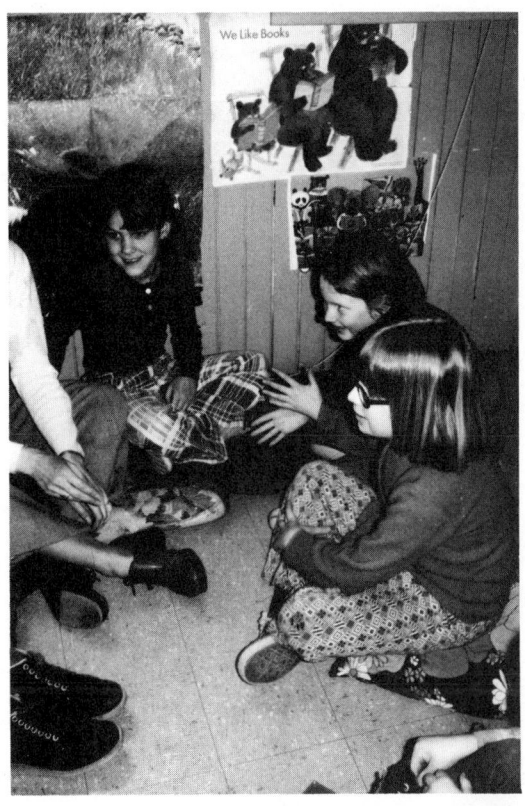

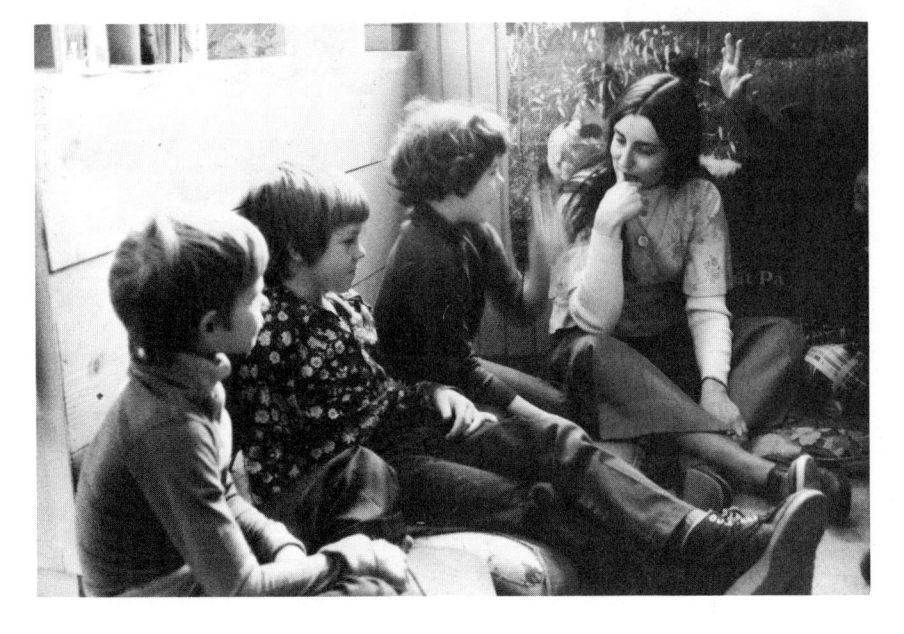

Photos by Sue B. Read

After a limited time of random moving and talking—ten minutes or so—ask everyone to choose a partner whom they will introduce to the whole class. Students should try to choose partners on the basis of some common interest they have noticed on their name tags. Ask them to try to choose someone whom they do not yet know.

Give partners six minutes to get to know one another in greater depth. Suggest that they take turns telling about themselves, starting with the information on the name tags.

Finally, have the entire class sit in a large circle, and give each person, one at a time, the chance to introduce his partner to the group. The introduction may include information from the name tag, as well as information learned from the one-to-one session.

Below is a name tag that was written out by one of the authors in an in-service workshop.

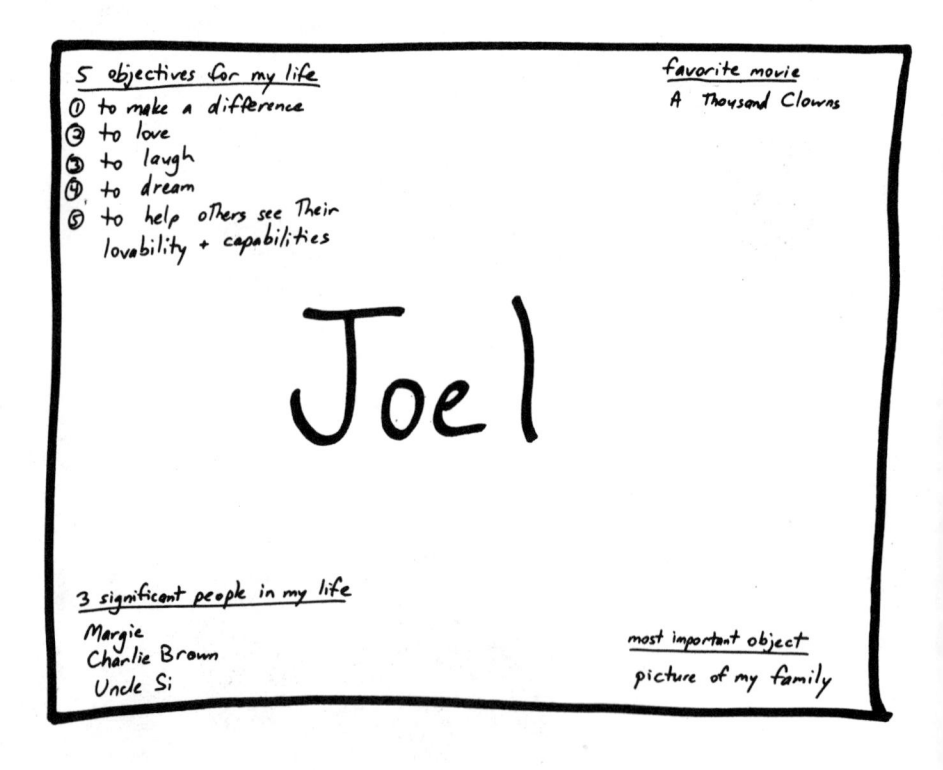

```
┌─────────────────────────────────────────────────────┐
│ 5 objectives for my life            favorite movie  │
│ ① to make a difference              A Thousand Clowns│
│ ② to love                                           │
│ ③ to laugh                                          │
│ ④ to dream                                          │
│ ⑤ to help others see their                          │
│    lovability + capabilities                        │
│                                                     │
│                                                     │
│                   Joel                              │
│                                                     │
│                                                     │
│                                                     │
│ 3 significant people in my life                     │
│   Margie                         most important object│
│   Charlie Brown                  picture of my family │
│   Uncle Si                                          │
└─────────────────────────────────────────────────────┘
```

EXERCISE: EMERGENCY NOW

The next exercise deals with a hypothetical situation: i. e. there is going to be a nuclear war. Only five persons will survive. Each survivor will be allowed to take five items into the underground city in which they will live for an extremely extended period of time. Food and clothing will be provided and need not be on anyone's list. The assignment for the students is: You have been chosen as one of the five survivors. You alone will pick the other four people who will also go to the underground city. Please list the four people in the world whom you would choose to go along with you. Also, please list five items that you would take along with you. We will make provisions to get any item into the underground city that you may want.

FOUR PEOPLE I WANT	FIVE ITEMS I WISH TO TAKE
_____	_____
_____	_____
_____	_____
_____	_____
	_____

1 *Can you share one reason for one choice that you have made above?*

2 *Do you see any illogical choices? Please describe:*

3 *What, if anything, did you learn from this exercise?*

Working through

Provide each student with an "Emergency Now" handout. Allow them three to five minutes to work on this exercise in a private place in the room; they may also be allowed to take this exercise home to work on there.

Once they have finished the exercise, have them gather small groups to share their answers to the situation. Point out the need for them to be as open and honest as possible. If you are working with very young children (ages six to ten), you may want to "work them through" the exercise. That is, you may need to read it to them (don't insist on correct spelling in the responses), or you may want to modify the exercise to fit your individual needs. This may include: your students not being able to read the instructions. So, read the instructions to them. Or, such statements as "What, if anything, did you learn from this exercise?" may be meaningless to your students. So, modify the statement. Example: "Did anyone else bring an item that you really liked and that you wished you had chosen?" You may also want to ask, "What was your last thought?" or "How did you feel about this exercise?"

We could go on and on. The point we are trying to make is that *you* can make all the difference in the "success" of any exercise. It is all in how you present, process, and conclude the exercise. Be understanding, gentle, and, most of all, nonjudgmental.

Finally, we have provided you with a few examples of this exercise.

EMERGENCY NOW

There is going to be a nuclear war. There will only be five survivors. Each survivor will be allowed to take five (5) items with them into the underground city in which they will live for a very extended period of time. Food and clothing will be provided and need not be on anyone's list. Now, this is your assignment: You have been chosen as one of the five survivors. You alone will pick the other four people who will also go to the underground city. Please list the four people in the world who you would chose to go along. Also, please list the five (5) items that you would take along with you. We will make provisions to get any item into the underground city that you may want.

Four people I want	Five items I wish to take
Mother	radio
boyfriend	shampoo
sister	brush
girlfriend	guitar
	diary/pen

Can you share one reason for one choice that you have made above: *girlfriend chosen for companionship, someone to talk to*

Do you see any illogical choices: Please describe: *shampoo-brush these aren't necessary, but desired.*

What, if anything, did you learn from this exercise: *I realized which people and things mean the most to me.*

EMERGENCY NOW

There is going to be a nuclear war. There will only be five survivors. Each survivor will be allowed to take five (5) items with them into the underground city in which they will live for a very extended period of time. Food and clothing will be provided and need not be on anyone's list. Now, this is your assignment: You have been chosen as one of the five survivors. You alone will pick the other four people who will also go to the underground city. Please list the four people in the world who you would chose to go along. Also, please list the five (5) items that you would take along with you. We will make provisions to get any item into the underground city that you may want.

Four people I want
- NURSE
- Rachel
- Wonder Woman
-

Five items I wish to take
- Laser Gun
- Car
- Survival Kit
- Stove
- Tool Box Full of tools

Can you share one reason for one choice that you have made above:

So we can build a colony

Do you see any illogical choices: Please describe:

No

What, if anything, did you learn from this exercise:

Survival

117 PROCESSING Chapter 7

There is going to be a nuclear war. There will only be five survivors. Each survivor will be allowed to take five (5) items with them into the underground city in which they will live for a very extended period of time. Food and clothing will be provided and need not be on anyone's list. Now, this is your assignment: You have been chosen as one of the five survivors. You alone will pick the other four people who will also go to the underground city. Please list the four people in the world who you would chose to go along. Also, please list the five (5) items that you would take along with you. We will make provisions to get any item into the underground city that you may want.

Four people I want	Five items I wish to take
Chan Colby	teddy bear
Mike Duby	shovle
Billy Canbury	gun wax-gun
Kelly Colby	book
	nickrascop

Can you share one reason for one choice that you have made above:

Chan to play with me!

Do you see any illogical choices: Please describe:

there all a.o.k.

What, if anything, did you learn from this exercise:

I love my teddy bear

EMERGENCY NOW

There is going to be a nuclear war. There will only be five survivors. Each survivor will be allowed to take five (5) items with them into the underground city in which they will live for a very extended period of time. Food and clothing will be provided and need not be on anyone's list. Now, this is your assignment: You have been chosen as one of the five survivors. You alone will pick the other four people who will also go to the underground city. Please list the four people in the world who you would chose to go along. Also, please list the five (5) items that you would take along with you. We will make provisions to get any item into the underground city that you may want.

Four people I want	Five items I wish to take
Kelly G.	Shuvles
thane H.	2 Books
holly L.	water
todd M.	Puzzlls
	A Game

Can you share one reason for one choice that you have made above:

A Shuvle to dig

Do you see any illogical choices: Please describe:

They are all ok.

What, if anything, did you learn from this exercise:

I coudnd live with oot Books

119 PROCESSING Chapter 7

EMERGENCY NOW

There is going to be a nuclear war. There will only be five survivors. Each survivor will be allowed to take five (5) items with them into the underground city in which they will live for a very extended period of time. Food and clothing will be provided and need not be on anyone's list. Now, this is your assignment: You have been chosen as one of the five survivors. You alone will pick the other four people who will also go to the underground city. Please list the four people in the world who you would chose to go along. Also, please list the five (5) items that you would take along with you. We will make provisions to get any item into the underground city that you may want.

Four people I want	Five items I wish to take
Mother	Minibike
Father	Television
Doctor Newhart	gasoline
~~list~~	Oil
friend	friend's minibike

Can you share one reason for one choice that you have made above:

I brought the doctor in case anybody was sick or hurt.

Do you see any illogical choices: Please describe:

NO

What, if anything, did you learn from this exercise:

nothing

120 HEALTH EDUCATION: THE SEARCH FOR VALUES

Photo by David M. Goodman

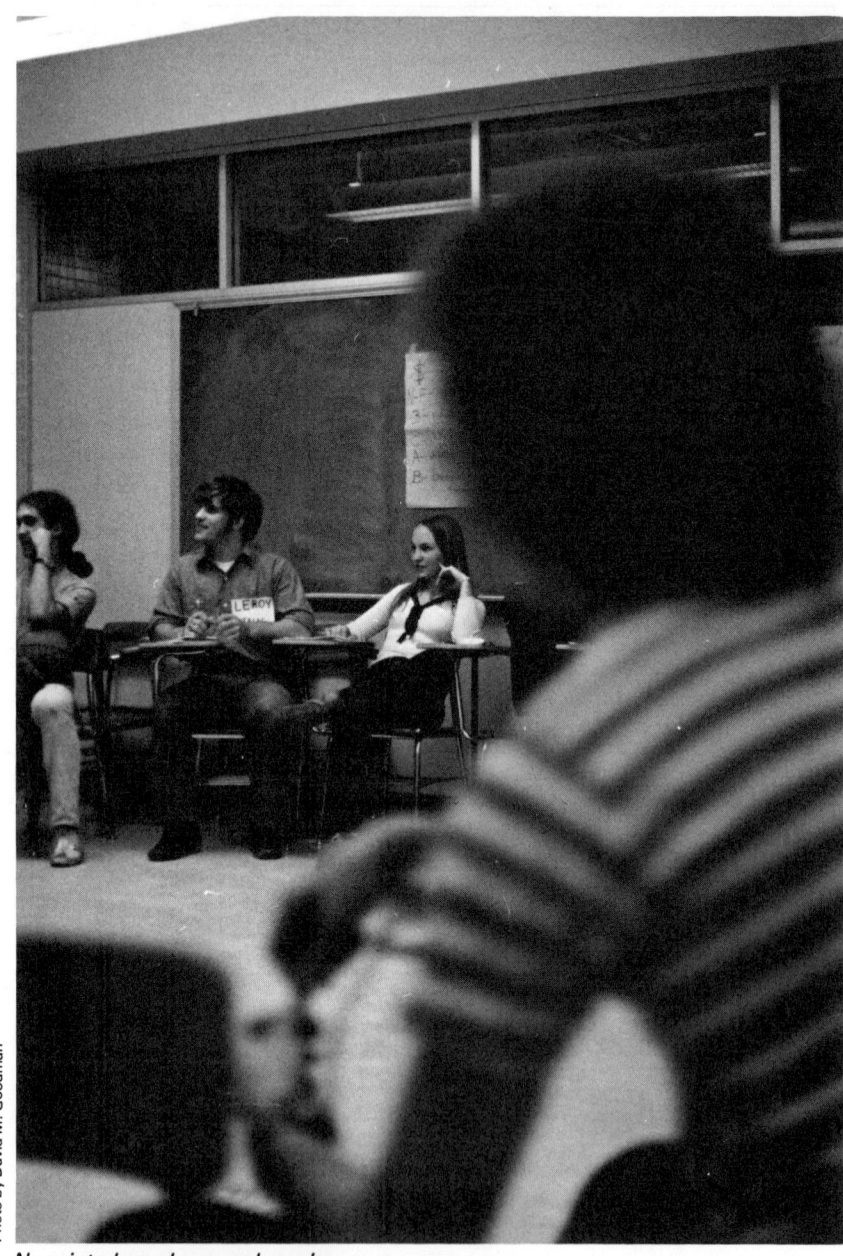

No printed word nor spoken plea
Can teach young minds what men should be,
Not all the books on all the shelves
But what the teachers are themselves. (Anonymous)

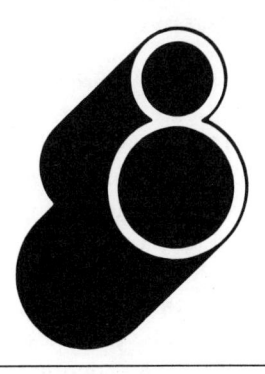

A HUMANISTIC APPROACH TO EVALUATION AND WAYS OF EVALUATING HUMANISTIC EDUCATION: COUNTING THE APPLES IN A SEED

This chapter could be subtitled "Evaluation: A Decision-making Tool for Students and Teachers." Not everyone sees evaluation in this light, however. To some people this concept is a threatening one, while others treat it lightly. For some it is necessary, while others avoid it at all costs. Depending on who is speaking, the concept is seen as both the future and the downfall of education.

These reactions intensify when we begin to think of evaluating humanistic or affective programs. John Goodlad (1966) speaks of an analogy that has implications for the evaluation of humanistic-education programs:

One does not often try to determine electrical current with a meter stick or lengths with an ammeter; we must be equally careful in trying to measure the successes of courses that differ in kind, rather than degree, by using a test intended for one as instrument to calibrate the other.

Or, to put it another way, it is not appropriate to use a stop watch or tape measure to evaluate diving, figure skating, and gymnastics, whereas it would be highly appropriate to use these means in evaluating a hundred-yard dash or a shot-put competition. We must stop using "the stop watch" in evaluating humanistic activities and outcomes.

However, working in a new and developing field, humanistic educators often find themselves at a loss for evaluation procedures that are both appropriate and effective. In this chapter, we offer some general guidelines as well as several specific activities that may be helpful in counting the apples in a seed (rather than counting the seeds in an apple).

GUIDELINES FOR HUMANISTIC EVALUATION

The purpose of evaluation, as we see it, is to provide data that will be helpful to the teacher and learner in making decisions. In this context, the purpose of evaluation is to improve the learning process, not necessarily to prove specific conclusions. Evaluation is decision-oriented rather than conclusion-oriented. Engaging students in evaluation procedures is a way of increasing their involvement, their feelings of power (that they do have some influence on what happens to them), as well as their feelings of responsibility. In this sense, evaluation can be an essential part of the learning process, rather than a block to it or a necessary evil.

Given the purpose of evaluation stated above, just what are its components? We use the following formula to illustrate this:

$$\text{Evaluation} = \text{Feedback} + \text{Feedforward}$$
$$= \text{Describe} + \text{Internalize} + \text{Prescribe}$$

Essentially, evaluation is an ongoing process of describing what has happened (what), noting the implications of what has happened (so what), and prescribing where/how to proceed (now what). The focus of the evaluation can be on the student's learning, the teacher's style, the teacher–student relationship, the curriculum, and/or on the classroom environment.

We have found a number of guidelines to be helpful in humanizing evaluation procedures. The list below is not meant to be all-inclusive— we encourage you to add your own ideas.

1 Many people have fears surrounding the whole notion of "evaluation." Many students equate evaluation with grading and all its negative side-effects (e.g. apple polishing, cramming, plagiarism,

cheating, tattling, vicious competition, focusing on "the grade" rather than on learning).[1] Many teachers equate evaluation with being judged, with having their jobs on the line. It is crucial for us to be sensitive to these kinds of feelings. It is also crucial for us to make clear the positive building purposes of evaluation before we engage in it. For instance, in asking students to provide their responses to a particular unit, we often preface the evaluation process with a statement of intent (e.g. "I am asking for your thoughts and reflections on this for two reasons: (1) to provide you with a chance to conceptualize, summarize, synthesize, inventory, or pull together your own experience and learnings; and (2) to provide you with an opportunity to give me ideas about how I can make the learning environment here better for all of us."). Evaluation can be a bridge (rather than an obstacle) between teacher and students.

2 It is extremely important that we orient our evaluations so that teachers and students can learn from their successes, as well as their "mistakes." Too often, evaluation is equated with "constructive" (alias "negative") criticism. We believe strongly that people learn best when they can build on their own strengths and successes, when they feel valuable. Let's focus on the "value" in evaluation. One simple (but not simplistic) example of this would be to ask students (and teacher) such questions as: "What was the high point for you in this unit?" "In looking at yourself over the past week, what is one thing that you appreciate about *you*?" "What is it that you think others in this class have appreciated about you and your behavior?" Evaluation can be used as a means to help students in validating themselves and others. If people are not "validated" (do not feel worthwhile, lovable, capable), then they become (emotional) in-valids. At first, students might feel a bit awkward in taking a positive focus in evaluation (because they've been brought up in a school system dominated by a "red-pencil mentality"), but over time, if done in a consistent manner, this positive orientation will take hold.

3 One reason why "evaluation" has always been so threatening is that often it is used only in a "terminal" fashion. The final exam at the end of the course leaves little room for either improvement or learning. We suggest that effective evaluation is both formative (the ongoing process of finding out where you are going while you are getting there) and summative (reflecting on where you have been once you have gotten there).

---

[1] Two excellent sources and resources in the area of grading are Howard Kirschenbaum, Sidney B. Simon, and Rodney Napier, *Wad-Ja-Get?: The Grading Game in American Education* (New York: Hart Publishing Co., Inc., 1971); and James Bellanca, Director, Center for Grading and Learning Alternatives, 811 Foxdale Road, Winnetka, Ill. 60093 (the Center conducts workshops and does consulting in the areas of grading alternatives, evaluation, and learning alternatives).

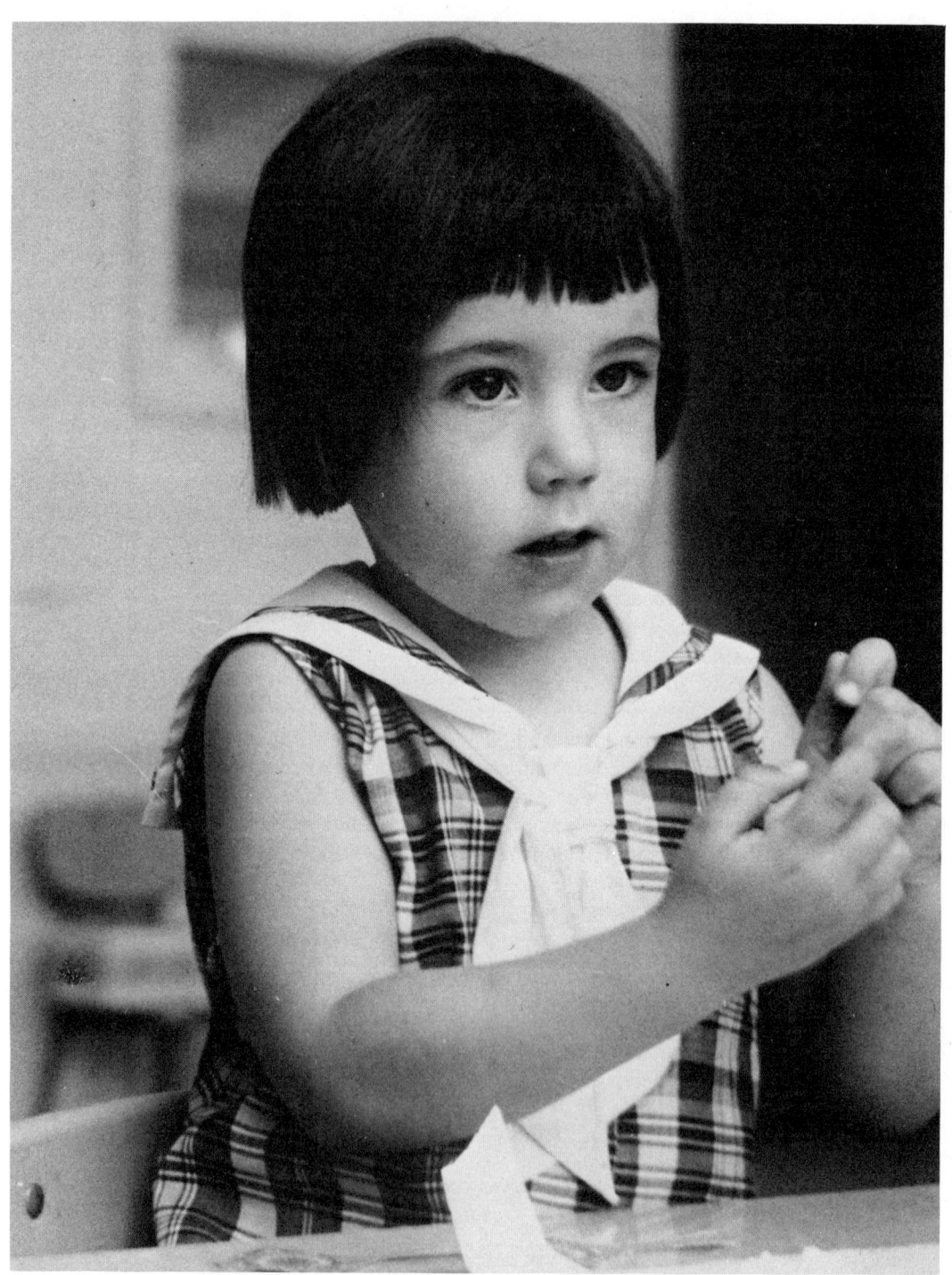

The mind of a child is a beautiful thing indeed. Feed it, nurture it, and allow it to grow freely.

4 No single evaluation mode will be one hundred per cent reliable or valid, nor will it speak to all students at all times. Hence, another evaluation principle emerges: We seek to be eclectic in terms of our evaluation methods. These methods can range from written to verbal, from obtrusive to unobtrusive, from self-generated data to data reported by observers. The evaluation processes described in the second half of this chapter reflect this range of methods.

5 Too often, evaluation methods only enhance convergent thinking (e.g. "When were the Prohibition laws passed?"), at the expense of divergent thinking (e.g. "What is the most important learning you have picked up from our unit on alcohol?"). Evaluation, if it is to be both effective and affective, must enhance both our convergent and divergent capacities.

6 In soliciting feedback from students, the teacher may find it helpful to keep these criteria in mind: Feedback is most helpful when: (a) it is descriptive rather than judgmental (e.g. "I noticed everyone laughed when you told your joke," rather than, "You weren't that funny today"); (b) it is specific rather than general (e.g. "I noticed that you only called on people who sit on the left side of the room," rather than, "You play favorites"); (c) it is directed toward changeable behaviors (e.g. "I noticed that you asked more questions than you made statements," rather than, "I think you nose is too big"); (d) it is solicited rather than imposed (this helps the receiver of the feedback "hear" it better); (e) it is well-timed (enhancing formative evaluation); and (f) it takes into account the needs of the receiver. These criteria encourage us to use feedback as "food for thought" rather than as "backbiting."

7 Alschuler and Ivey (1973) offer some guidelines that are helpful in evaluating the long-term internalization of humanistic attitudes and skills. They suggest five kinds of questions that can aid teachers and students in assessing the effectiveness of humanistic activities and curricula: (a) Did the student *attend* to the activity presented?; (b) did the student thoroughly *experience* what is to be learned?; (c) did the individual clearly *conceptualize* the experience?; (d) did the person *relate* the experience to other important aspects of his or her life?; and (e) did the student *use* or act on the learning provided? By the way, these five questions can serve as a logical and psychological format for sequencing humanistic activities. Educators might find it beneficial to weave questions of this nature throughout their evaluations of humanistic curricula.

EVALUATION ACTIVITIES: A BAKER'S DOZEN

What can the teacher do that is realistic and practical to implement the guidelines just stated? What follows is a baker's dozen of ways of gathering evaluation data in the classroom. You may want to modify these ideas because of your particular students' age, maturity, and experience in being part of the evaluation process.

1 Feedforward form

At the beginning of a semester, or periodically throughout the year, you may obtain some important information from your students by having them respond to questions (verbally and/or in writing) about their needs, hopes, expectations, and learning styles. A positive consequence of this activity is that students will also have a chance to increase their achievement motivation by focusing on their goals and looking for ways of reaching them. Here are some questions for you and your students to chew on (you will probably want to generate your own, too):

a What are your reasons for taking this course?
b How would you like this course to be run and what would you like your part to be in helping the class to function in this manner?
c What do you expect from the teacher?
d What do you expect from yourself?
e What do you expect from the other members of the class?
f What special concerns, issues, or questions would you like to have as part of the agenda of this class?
g What do you not want from this class?
h How would you describe your own learning style: How, where, when, and with whom do you learn best?
i What do you hope to accomplish as a result of participating in this class?

The feedforward form can serve as an important diagnostic tool and as a springboard for mutual goal-setting between teacher and students. There are a number of ways to follow up this initial diagnosis. For example, the teacher can also respond to the questions and respond to such questions as: "How would you describe your own teaching style: How, where, when, and with whom . . . ?" After comparing his/her responses with the students' answers, the teacher could then identify structures that might help maximize the strengths of each. Another option is to have the students brainstorm the structures (e.g. guidelines, rules, timelines, curriculum topics) that would help them build on (or experiment with) their learning styles and interests. As a way of formalizing this, the students can then develop self-contracts, as well as a contract with the teacher.

2 "Dear Me" letter

This evaluation instrument is excellent for gathering student-generated data. It can be used almost anytime—at the end of the day, at the end of a unit, at the end of a semester. Essentially, students take time to reflect on their experiences, and to conceptualize, relate, and apply their learnings. The teacher supplies each student with a sheet of carbon paper. The student can then turn the carbon copy in to the teacher and keep the original in an ongoing class journal. The evaluation data can prove to be as valuable to the student as it is to the teacher (especially if kept in a cumulative format, as in a journal). It is helpful to include in the "Dear Me" letter questions that are both convergent and open-ended. In order to minimize "psyching out" the teacher, it would probably also be helpful to allow students to respond anonymously, if they so choose. Here are some sample questions to which students can respond in their "Dear Me" letters:

a The high point of the class/unit for me was . . .
b I learned that I . . . [relearned . . . became aware of . . . noticed . . .]
c One thing I liked about my own behavior was . . .
d One thing I appreciated about the teacher's behavior was . . .
e The most useful idea or learning for me was . . .
f One change I would recommend is . . .
g One way I have used or applied a learning from this class is . . .
h I hope . . .
i I wonder . . .
j I'm proud that I . . .
k A challenge or obstacle I face . . .
l As I look back on this class/unit, four feelings that come to me are . . .
m I feel most lovable and capable in this class when . . .
n I enjoyed . . .
o This week, I was like a [metaphor] because . . .
p Some factors in this class that have been helping me to learn are . . .
q Some factors in this class that have blocked my learning are . . .
r A contract I want to make with myself/the teacher/my classmates is . . .
s I am looking forward to . . .
t The most valuable thing for me . . .
u This makes me think about . . .
v Today I have . . .
w One thing I appreciated about my classmates is . . .
x If I were the teacher . . .
y Open comment . . .

Here are some additional ways of using "Dear Me" letters in the classroom: (1) For any one letter, it would probably be best to have six or less questions. The teacher may choose to have the same questions in each "Dear Me" letter, or to offer some variety (we've found that this often helps to maintain the students' attention). The letters should be spaced over a semester's time, perhaps one every third week. We encourage you to generate questions of your own, and to ask the students for their ideas as well. (2) You may want to use some of the sentence stems just given in other ways and at other times. For instance, the students could do a "whip"—each person who wanted a turn (the right to pass would hold here) could share aloud his/her response to one of the sentence stems. This could lead into a class discussion, if appropriate. Or, the teacher may want to use the sentence stems given above in feedforward forms. (3) One way of starting a new day/unit/week is for the teacher to read anonymous excerpts from students' "Dear Me" letters. This can serve the three-fold purpose of letting the students know that the teacher has read and responded to their thoughts; providing a bridge between the previous day/unit/week and the upcoming one; and helping students to see that they are not "alone" (that other people have similar thoughts, feelings, and reactions), that they are not "weird." In order to protect the confidentiality of individual responses, the teacher may ask students to note at the top of their Dear Me letters an *R* (read) or *DR* (don't read to the class).

3 Defuzzing wheel

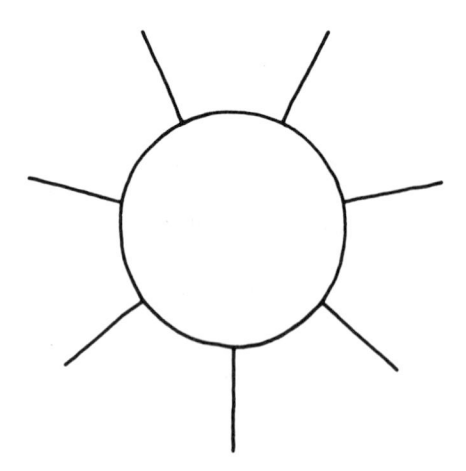

This is a very flexible tool that can be used to generate either feedforward or feedback data. Here's how it works: Ask your students to draw a circle with numerous spokes radiating from it. Next, ask the students to place in the center of the circle the "fuzzy concept" to be defuzzed. For example, at the beginning, middle, and end of a unit on alcoholism, or at all three points, you might ask students to defuzz the concept "alcoholic." Or, if you were studying the Revolutionary War, you could ask students to defuzz "George Washington." Or, if you were doing a unit on nutrition, your students could defuzz the concept "good diet." The process of defuzzing involves the students in brainstorming and freely associating everything they know or connect with the concept to be defuzzed. Students take some time by themselves to complete their defuzzing wheels by placing their ideas on the spokes radiating from the circle. These ideas could take the form of single words (e.g. for "George Washington": President, general, honest); phrases (e.g. for "George Washington": led our country in the Revolutionary War, "Father" of our country, lived at Mount Vernon); or pictures drawn by the students or cut from magazines (e.g. for "George Washington": a picture of the

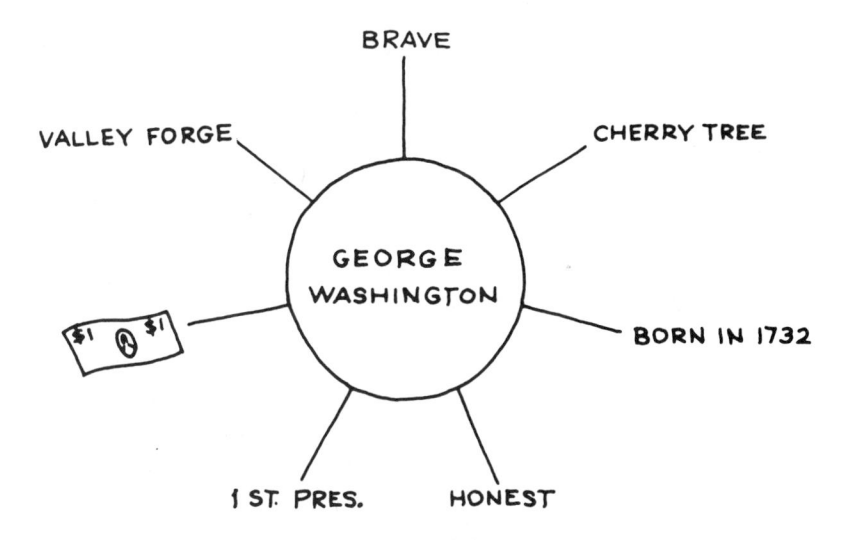

dollar bill, a picture of the White House, a picture of Washington crossing the Delaware).

After students have had a chance to complete their wheels individually, it is often helpful to have them form small groups and share their ideas. This sharing has several benefits: It provides an opportunity for students to "cross fertilize"—to engage in a peer-teaching situation; it encourages divergent thinking; and it allows students to expand their original lists.

Following this sharing, we like to give students a chance to do some individual reflecting. This can be facilitated by having students "code" their defuzzing wheels (e.g. circle the idea that you most strongly associate with the fuzzy concept; underline the ideas about which you would like to learn more; put a question mark next to those ideas about which you have some doubts; place a *T* next to those ideas about which you would be willing to teach your classmates; mark an *R* next to those ideas for which you might be willing to write a report). The teacher may want to have students verbally report on some of their codings and/or to turn in their findings in writing. If done at the beginning of a unit, this would enable both the students and teacher to ascertain interests, skills, and possible directions. If done in the middle of a unit, it would provide valuable feedback for the class on next steps. If done at the end of a unit, it could serve as a time for the students to conceptualize their learnings and for the teacher to assess the effect and impact of the unit.

4 Whatcha know, whatcha need to know

This is a "cousin" of the defuzzing wheel, and can be used at the beginning, middle, and/or end of a unit/day/week. Ask your students to draw three columns on a sheet of paper, with the following headings: What I Know; What I Need to Know; Possible Resources. After they have a topic in mind (e.g. "George Washington," or "good diet"), they can proceed to brainstorm their responses under each of the three headings. As with the defuzzing wheel, next steps could include sharing in small groups and individual reflection (e.g. using codings . . . put an *I* next to those topics and ideas for which you would like to be in an interest group with some of your classmates; place an *F* next to those items on which you would like us to focus (more) time during this unit).

The class can springboard off this inventory by forming interest groups or work groups around particular topics (in effect, students have a chance to generate part of their curriculum and to structure part of the learning environment). This technique might also allow the teacher a chance to encourage students to support and teach each other (e.g. by having a student who knows something about the topic "teach" it to a student who had the topic listed in the "Need to Know" column). As with the defuzzing wheel, this activity can generate data for both feedforward and feedback.

5 Rank-ordering

In addition to helping students clarify their values and develop decision-making skill, rank-ordering can be used to help them in the evaluation process. The teacher and students need only generate rankings related to the classroom environment, the curriculum, student learning, and teacher behavior. Here are some sample rankings. We hope these will stimulate your thinking.

a   I would most like to write a report on: alcoholism; the laws regarding marijuana; the effects of cigarette smoking.
b   Today, I am feeling most like a: bubbling brook; calm lake; swamp.
c   What I like about our classroom: the seating arrangement; the amount of homework; the degree of informality.
d   In the unit we just completed, the teacher reminded me of a: wishbone; backbone; jawbone; hambone; trombone.
e   If I were the teacher, I would: do more lecturing; do less lecturing; do about the same amount of lecturing.
f   The most important part of the last unit was: learning about the dietary habits of other cultures; learning about the basic food groups; talking about our own eating habits.
g   What I value in a classroom: chances for self-direction; time to work in small groups; guest speakers.
h   What I like about our classroom: the humor; the orderliness; the caring.

As with other evaluation activities, you and your students may find it helpful to follow a sequence of individual reflection— small-group sharing—individual reflection—report out in the large group (or to the teacher). This allows room for the individual student, the class, and the teacher to make evaluation decisions based on the data generated through the rank-ordering process.

6 Continuum

The continuum is another values-clarification strategy that can be employed as an evaluating strategy. Teacher and students can respond to such continua as:

a   In this class, I feel: powerful———powerless.
b   For me, the last unit we covered was: new———old hat.
c   I feel that the other students in this class are: accepting———unaccepting.
d   While in class this week, I have felt: excited———bored.
e   In looking at my own efforts in this class, I am feeling supersatisfied———downright dissatisfied.
f   In my relationship with the teacher, I've been feeling very close———very distant.
g   During the past week, I've learned a lot———learned nothing.

The continuum, like the rank order, can be an excellent starting point for further discussion and exploration. For example, you may want to use it as a stimulus for goal-setting: In that case, ask the students to note where they are *now* on the continuum, then ask them to place another mark at the point where they would like to be at the end of a specific time period (e.g. two weeks, end of the unit, and so on). This helps students to note the difference or similarity between what they would *like* to do and what they are *likely* to do. From this awareness can emerge the motivation for goal-setting (e.g. "What could you do and/or what can the teacher do to make this class more satisfying for you?"). Here, the teacher can be most helpful by supporting the student in identifying specific next steps in reaching the goal (e.g. "I want you to call on me as least once during each class," "I want to write a report on child-rearing practices in other countries," "I want a chance to work with Bill in an interest group").

7 Voting questions

Here is yet another values-clarification activity that can be used as an evaluation strategy. It is a strategy that can be used very quickly and effectively on the spur of the moment to assess "where the students are at." Over time, students will have learned the voting hand signals: rotating the arm vigorously with the thumb up = strongly agree; holding the arm with the thumb up = agree; holding the arm with the thumb down = disagree; pumping the arm with the thumb down = strongly disagree; folding arms = pass option. Each voting question starts with the words "How many of you . . .?" Here are some samples to whet your appetite:

How many of you . . .

a Came from an enjoyable class last period?
b Are hungry?
c Found the homework to be hard?
d Want to spend more time working on our present unit?
e Find our textbook to be helpful in explaining concepts?
f Want to take a five-minute stretch break now?
g Would like to form interest groups when we come to the unit on environmental education?
h Think we should invite more guest speakers to the class?

There are a number of ways to use voting questions. Some teachers find them helpful as a "break" in and of themselves; they tend to grab the students' attention and help to change the pace. Some teachers use them spontaneously when they do not have a clear reading of their class's energy or interest levels (or when there seems to be a split of opinion or interest in the class). Other teachers consciously build in no more than five voting questions at the start of each class. Voting questions can either stand by themselves (with the teacher and students filing the results away in their minds) or can lead later to teacher–student conferences, or can be a stimulus for a class discussion. Or all three— that's the beauty of these activities—you can choose flexibly what is most appropriate for the situation.

133 A HUMANISTIC APPROACH TO EVALUATION   Chapter 8

8 Coat of arms

This activity offers students a chance to generate evaluation data through a nonverbal medium. It is crucial for the teacher to emphasize the fact that this is not an art contest—as long as the student knows what his/her drawings mean, that's all that is important.

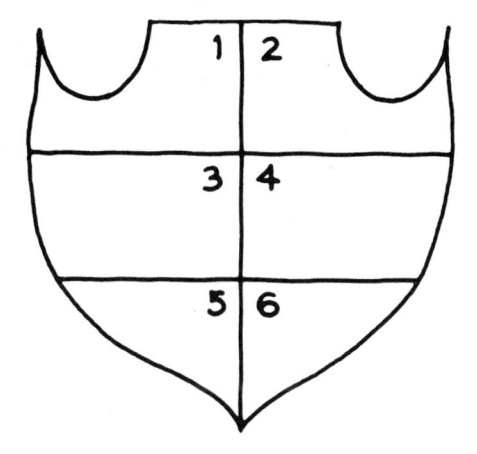

You can start this off by mentioning to the students that in days of old, when knights were bold, many people had their own coat of arms, which reflected their background, beliefs, and dreams. This is an opportunity for the class members to create their own coats of arms. Ask each student to draw a six-section shield on a full sheet of paper (some teachers have students use big, bright sheets of construction paper). For each of the six sections, the teacher offers a question to which the students respond (using pictures and symbols, but no words). Here are some sample questions that could help students evaluate their class experience:

a Can you draw a picture(s) or symbol(s) that represents the way in which you see yourself in this class?
b What picture or symbol can you use to reflect the way in which your classmates see you?
c How do you think the teacher sees you?
d How about a picture to represent one or more of your strengths as a student in this class? Allow yourself the luxury of bragging just for a moment.
e What is one thing you would like to get better at as a student?
f In looking at our class, what do you see as its greatest strength?
g In looking at our class, what do you perceive to be its greatest concern (what do we need to work on more?)?
h How would you like to describe yourself at the end of this semester?
i How would you like the teacher to see you at the end of this semester?
j If you were the teacher . . .
k What are you most proud about in this class?

Of course, you need not lock yourself into six sections; at times, you might choose to use fewer or more. At times, you might also want to have some magazines available—students can make a collage coat of arms by cutting out appropriate pictures in response to the questions.

There are innumerable ways to follow up the coat-of-arms activity. In an atmosphere of safety (where there are no killer phrases or put-downs of each other's pictures), students enjoy sharing their inevitably creative drawings with their peers. This sharing can occur in a combination of modes: talking in pairs or trios, having volunteers talk about their coats of arms before the whole class, setting up a "whip" (where each student who so wished could talk briefly about his/her coat of arms), and/or creating a "gallery walk" (posting the shields on the wall or bulletin board—students gather around them at their own pace as if in a museum). As with other values-clarification and evaluation activities, it is important for the teacher to participate in this, too—you can post your coat of arms with the others in the gallery.

The teacher may choose to go beyond the self-evaluation steps listed above by engaging each student in a private conference (which could lead to goal-setting as with the continuum) and/or by meeting with small groups of students to analyze/synthesize the evaluation data that has been generated. You and your students might consider repeating the coat of arms activity several times during the course of the year. You'll probably find much fascinating longitudinal evaluation data with which to work, investigate feelings, investigate self, etc.

9 Observation

Usually, this word strikes fear in the hearts and minds of those being observed. Often, a salary increase, tenure, or, at the very least, one's self-esteem are at stake. It doesn't have to be this way—observation can be a highly positive and powerful evaluation mode. How so? By creating a situation that is safe for the person being observed. How to do that? By following the feedback guidelines mentioned earlier in this chapter.

You might consider asking one of your students, a friend from outside school, or a colleague who has a free period to serve periodically as an observer. You have control over what role the observer takes— ranging from someone who keeps his/her eyes open to anything and everything in the classroom to someone who focuses on a specific goal, objective, area that you identify. An example of the latter role would be the observer who tallies the number of times the teacher asks narrow questions, asks broad questions, gives information, gives an opinion, gives a direction during one class period. Or, if the teacher is interested in other classroom variables, he/she might ask the observer to keep track of the amount of time the teacher is talking during a class, the amount of time students are talking, or the percentage of class time during which the students are working individually, the students are working in small groups, the students are discussing in the whole group, the teacher is giving a lecture.

Here, the important point is for the teacher to "take charge" by sharing the feedback criteria with the observer at the start and by defining the observer's role in a way that would be most helpful to the teacher. Essentially, the question to ask is: What data would be most helpful to me in making decisions about the direction of the class, my behavior, my relationship with the students?

10 "Dear Teacher" letter

Meet the "Dear Me" letter's first cousin. You can tell them apart by noting these characteristics: (a) Obviously, the "Dear Teacher" letter is addressed to the teacher, whereas the "Dear Me" letter is addressed to the student; (b) the "Dear Teacher" letter is more open-ended than its cousin, in that there are no sentence stems to which the students respond—rather, this is a chance for them to make note of whatever is on their mind and in their hearts. Other than these differences, the "Dear Teacher" letter may be used, adapted, and followed up in the same ways as the "Dear Me" letter.

11 Standardized instruments

The standardized instrument is a potentially rich resource for gathering evaluation data. There are hundreds of instruments that have been developed to gather data on such areas as teacher behavior, teacher attitudes, student behavior, student attitudes, teacher-student relationships, student-student relationships, classroom morale, and leadership styles.[2]

We offer these considerations for when and if you choose to use a standardized instrument to gather evaluation data: (a) We encourage you to modify and adapt these instruments, just as you would modify and adapt any of the preceding evaluation methods. It is crucial that the evaluation instrument be one that speaks to your and your students' needs and goals. Far too many people just pluck an instrument off the shelf and administer it blindly. (b) While using or adapting the instrument, it would be helpful if the teacher reiterated its purpose as a positive, growth-oriented evaluation tool, rather than as a device that would be grading or degrading the students. Far too many of us have had distressing experiences with standardized tests; we need to be

---

[2]For references to and samples of some of these instruments, see J. William Pfeiffer and Richard Heslin, *Instrumentation in Human Relations Training*; N.L. Gage, *Handbook of Research on Teaching*; Robert Sinclair, *Elementary School Environment Survey*; and Warren Lacefield and Henry P. Cole, *Educational Preference Scale*.

sensitive to this possibility if we choose to use them. (c) In this line, it is important to think through how the data should or could be used after it is collected; our bias is to use it in a descriptive way (for decision-making), rather than in a restrictive way (for categorizing students).

12 New and good calendar

As mentioned early in this chapter, we firmly believe that people can learn from their successes (as well as from their "mistakes"). Furthermore, we believe that teachers can learn from their successes (our observation is that teachers often receive more flak than plaques). The first step in such learning is to identify those successes.

Making a "New and Good Calendar" is a simple activity that encourages teachers to give themselves a little credit and to counter the red-pencil mentality that has permeated the thinking of so many of us. The calendar invites the teacher on a daily basis to note what was "new and good" in school (or, if really ambitious, in each class). You could enter items ranging from major, public victories (e.g. "I was praised by three parents for helping their children," "I received tenure," "The students in fifth period gave me a surprise party") to major, private victories (e.g. "John took an interest in the class for the first time," "Gail felt enough trust in me to want to talk with me after school," "I felt so good about the way in which I spontaneously changed gears during third period today").

At first glance, this activity might appear trivial. Nonetheless, it carries with it several important messages: (a) The teacher is a legitimate and crucial source of evaluation data, (b) There are positive, growthful, successful happenings in each and every class, even those that the teacher thinks have "bombed." It's just a matter of orienting ourselves and practicing looking for them; (c) The teacher is a human being, with needs, hopes, skills, concerns, and strengths. We need to acknowledge this and to let the air out of the "closet syndrome" (witness the fact that many students think that the teacher goes into the closet at the end of the school day and then re-emerges the next morning—e.g. note the surprise on students' faces when they see their teachers at the grocery store); (d) If such a calendar is maintained over an extended period, we are convinced that a number of positive patterns will emerge for the teacher. Once these are identified, the teacher can be more conscious and conscientious about building on them. And that, for us, is what evaluation is all about—a process for building, not for tearing down.

13 The "nice things box"

This delicious treat is a good way to bring our baker's dozen to a close. We have all heard of the suggestion box. Most of us probably envision a little-used box tucked away in a corner of an office or teachers' lounge. And our impression or experience is that when the suggestion box is used, it is often an anonymous crank note that is received.

In contrast, we envision the Nice Things Box as a potentially much-used, personal, and positive approach to generating and sharing evaluation data. It is based on several principles: (1) Students (as well as teachers) have strengths that can be identified and maximized. (2) The evaluation process need not be limited to teacher-student interaction. This activity provides a way for students to share evaluation information with each other. (3) By acknowledging each other's strengths and successes, the teacher and the students will increase the strength and probability of success in developing a sense of community in the classroom. These principles all serve to make evaluation a growthful process rather than a threatening one.

You might find it helpful to introduce this activity by puncturing the myth around the old jingle, "Sticks and stones will break my bones, but names will never hurt me." It just ain't so.[3] A class discussion and individual reflection on the effects of put-downs, as well as on ways of giving supportive feedback to each other, might be a good starter.

Then, place a box in the classroom and establish the following guidelines: (a) Anyone may at any time put a "nice thing" in the box, (b) This "nice thing" (feel free to call it whatever you and your students want—some people like to call them "warm fuzzies") would be an honest, positive statement about another individual(s) in the class (e.g. "Dear Frank—I liked the points you made during our discussion yesterday," "Hi, Betty—I appreciate the fact that you were concerned with how I was feeling yesterday," "Dear Mr. Green—Thanks for being so patient with me on our term paper") (c) You may choose whether or not to sign your name to the statement, (d) Periodically, the teacher or a student (on a rotating basis) can "deliver" the messages/massages.

If carried on consistently and over time, this activity can help students to take responsibility for part of the evaluation process. The class may choose to springboard off the "nice things" box and set up a more public "nice things" bulletin board, validation circles (e.g. 5 minutes at the end of each day to share verbally appreciations for each other in a public forum), or special-person days (e.g. on a rotating basis, each person in the class would be the "focus person" and would receive 5 minutes of positive evaluation data from his/her peers and teacher).

---

[3]See Sidney B. Simon, *I Am Loveable and Capable*—the "IALAC" story—available from the National Humanistic Education Center, 110 Spring St., Saratoga Springs, N.Y. 12866.

A QUICK SUMMARY AND A REQUEST FOR FEEDBACK

In this chapter, we have set out a definition for "evaluation," and noted some of the guidelines underlying a humanistic approach to evaluation and approaches to evaluating humanistic education. What followed was a baker's-dozen inventory of evaluation tools that can be used in the classroom.

In an attempt to "practice what we teach," we would like to close this chapter by asking you to give us feedback on the book. We have a strong commitment to be of service and support to teachers and students and would like your help in improving our product. We encourage you to choose one or more of the evaluation tools presented in this chapter (or one of your own), and use it in evaluating this book. Please send your feedback to Dr. Joel Goodman, National Humanistic Education Center, 110 Spring Street, Saratoga Springs, N.Y. 12866, or to Dr. Don Read, Butterhill Road, Amherst, Ma. 01002. Thanks in advance for your help on this!

REFERENCES

Alschuler, Alfred, and Ivey, Allen. "Internalization: The Outcome of Psychological Education," *Personnel and Guidance Journal* (May 1973): 607-10.

Gage, N. L. *Handbook of Research on Teaching.* Chicago: Rand McNally and Co., 1963.

Goodlad, John. *The Changing School Curriculum.* New York: Fund for the Advancement of Education, 1966.

Goodman, Joel B. "The Development, Implementation, and Evaluation of a Humanistic Process Education Program." Doctoral dissertation, University of Massachusetts, 1974.

Hawley, Robert C., and Hawley, Isabel L. *Developing Human Potential.* Amherst, Mass.: ERA Press, 1975, pp. 22-23.

Hutchinson, Thomas. "Some Overlooked Implications of Purpose: To Provide Data for Decision Making." Paper presented at A.E.R.A., Chicago, Ill., 1972.

Lacefield, Warren, and Cole, Henry P. Educational Preference Scale. Lexington: University of Kentucky, 1972.

Morra, Frank. " A Practical Approach to Measurement." Unpublished paper, University of Virginia Evaluation Research Center, 1973.

_____, Frank. "A Survey of Instruments Which May Be Used in the Assessment of Teachers." Unpublished paper, University of Virginia Evaluation Research Center, 1973.

Pfeiffer, J. William, and Heslin, Richard. *Instrumentation in Human Relations Training*. Iowa City, Iowa: University Associates, 1973.

Scriven, Michael. "Pros and Cons about Goal-Free Evaluation," *Evaluation Comment* (December 1972): 1-4.

Sinclair, Robert L. *Elementary School Environment Survey*. Amherst, Mass.: University of Massachusetts, 1969.

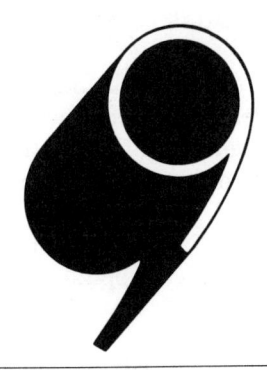

A FINAL NOTE

Once there was a toad who lived in a swamp. The grown-up toads at this swamp would push the toad around. The toad didn't like this treatment but his mommy and daddy told him that this was good. Once the toad was sent to a nearby co-operative swamp to stay for the summer. At this swamp the grown-up toads didn't push him around. He had fun and was freer than ever before. The toads here taught him how to be free but not how to be happy when he wasn't free. When he got back to his home swamp the grown-up toads started to push him around again, but now he wanted to be free. He didn't listen to the grown-up toads and he was killed. Back at the nearby co-operative swamp the toads were real happy because they had given the little visitor a happy time, a new experience, and a taste of freedom.[1]

The parable presented above may ring painfully true to many people who have participated in a values-clarification workshop or have read values-clarification books. One often takes away from such an experience a great deal of excitement and hope. Unfortunately, the "real world" does not always welcome this excitement and hope. Fellow teachers and administrators may feel threatened by new ideas, students may become puzzled by a new orientation, and you may become disheartened by the roadblocks you encounter.

[1] Terry Borton, *Reach, Touch, and Teach* (New York: McGraw-Hill Book Co., 1970, p. 70).

142 HEALTH EDUCATION: THE SEARCH FOR VALUES

We have a strong and serious commitment to helping you, the reader, to use and to adapt the ideas in this book without meeting the same figurative fate as our little toad. We offer the following guidelines on how to get started, based on our own experience and on the experience of thousands of teachers. Of course, not all the ideas listed below will apply to your situation. In fact, having an awareness of this is the first guideline. But many of them will apply—and we hope that you find them to be supportive "training wheels" . . . ride on!

2 Remember that values clarification is an *ongoing process*—don't expect to flick a magic wand and find a panacea.

3 In the same light, be(a)ware of others who expect values clarification to be a cure-all. This often manifests itself when they are disappointed that values clarification used in a health course didn't "cure" the school's "drug problem" in one semester. Values clarification is a preventive approach—not a Band-Aid.

4 Try to create a safe classroom environment, one in which students (and teacher) have a right to pass (it is crucial that we respect others' space and privacy), one in which their statements are accepted. Try to avoid moralizing, and imposing or deposing others' values. Attempt to expose your values whenever appropriate.

5 Try to experience values clarification as much as possible yourself, by participating in workshops, reading, and participating in activities in the classroom along with the students.

6 Start by using values activities, clarifying responses, and third-level lessons with which you feel comfortable. Be flexible—there is no one recipe for being a values-clarification facilitator. In fact, as Verta Mae says:

And when I cook, I never measure or weigh anything. I cook by vibration. I can tell by the look and smell of it. Most of the ingredients in this book are approximate. Some of the recipes that people gave me list the amounts, but for my part, I just do it by vibration. Different strokes for different folks. Do your thing your way . . .[2]

7 Remember that values clarification can be fun, but that it is not for fun. Other people in your environment may not have this perspective—you may choose to communicate it to them in some way.

8 Try to diagnose the students' needs and interests—build your activities and lessons to speak to them. Later on, call upon the students to help generate new strategies. Ultimately, it would be wonderful for the students to have an active part in developing their own emerging curriculum.

[2] Excerpt from *Vibration Cooking* by Verta Mae. © 1970 by Verta Grosvenor. Reprinted by permission of Doubleday & Company, Inc.

9 Continually examine your role and values as a teacher—this is crucial, both in terms of your personal growth and your professional development.

10 Focus your curriculum on the development of the cognitive, affective, active, and interpersonal skills enumerated in chapter 2. In this way, the activities, clarifying responses, and third-level lessons will be given direction and purpose. In fact, many teachers use the skills to delineate their curriculum objectives.

11 Beware of the effects of grades and avoid grading students on "their values."[3]

12 Start with lower-risk activities. Provide opportunities for differing levels of risk. Alternate the arenas in which participation occurs (e.g. individual reflection, small-group sharing, large-group sharing).

13 Be ready to express what values clarification is *not*, since it often has some strong (and inaccurate) connotations. For instance, values clarification is *not*: sensitivity training (values clarification has safety guidelines in its process—e.g. the right to pass); therapy (although it may be therapeutic in a sense); a collection of gimmicks, fun and games (again, it may be fun, but it is not *for* fun); behavior modification (in fact, values clarification is at the other end of the continuum—it seeks to help people internalize the locus of decision-making); a space-killer, time-killer (it is not to be used only to "fill in" the five minutes before the bell rings or to use on the day before vacation because the students won't do anything else).

14 Establish the norm of unfinished business in the classroom; there may be times when students feel as if they have not completed their reflection or sharing around a particular values issue. You may want to suggest that they take responsibility for themselves and identify a time, place, and way in which they would like to bring closure (e.g. outside of class, in class the next day).

15 Encourage students keep an ongoing class journal (which is private). This can help them (and you, if they choose to share it with you) inventory their growth over time and note the cumulative effects of the values-clarification approach.

16 Solicit feedback and feedforward (evaluation). See chapter 8 for in-depth ideas on how to do this.

17 Initially, you may find security in drawing from the multitude of structured values-clarification activities. But try to wean yourself away from these; develop your own activities, move towards spontaneity, and avoid falling into the "humanistic technician" trap (of "cranking" students through exercises).

---

[3]See Howard Kirschenbaum, Sidney B. Simon, and Rodney W. Napier, *Wad-Ja-Get?*. New York: Hart Publishing Co., 1971.

No Words Needed

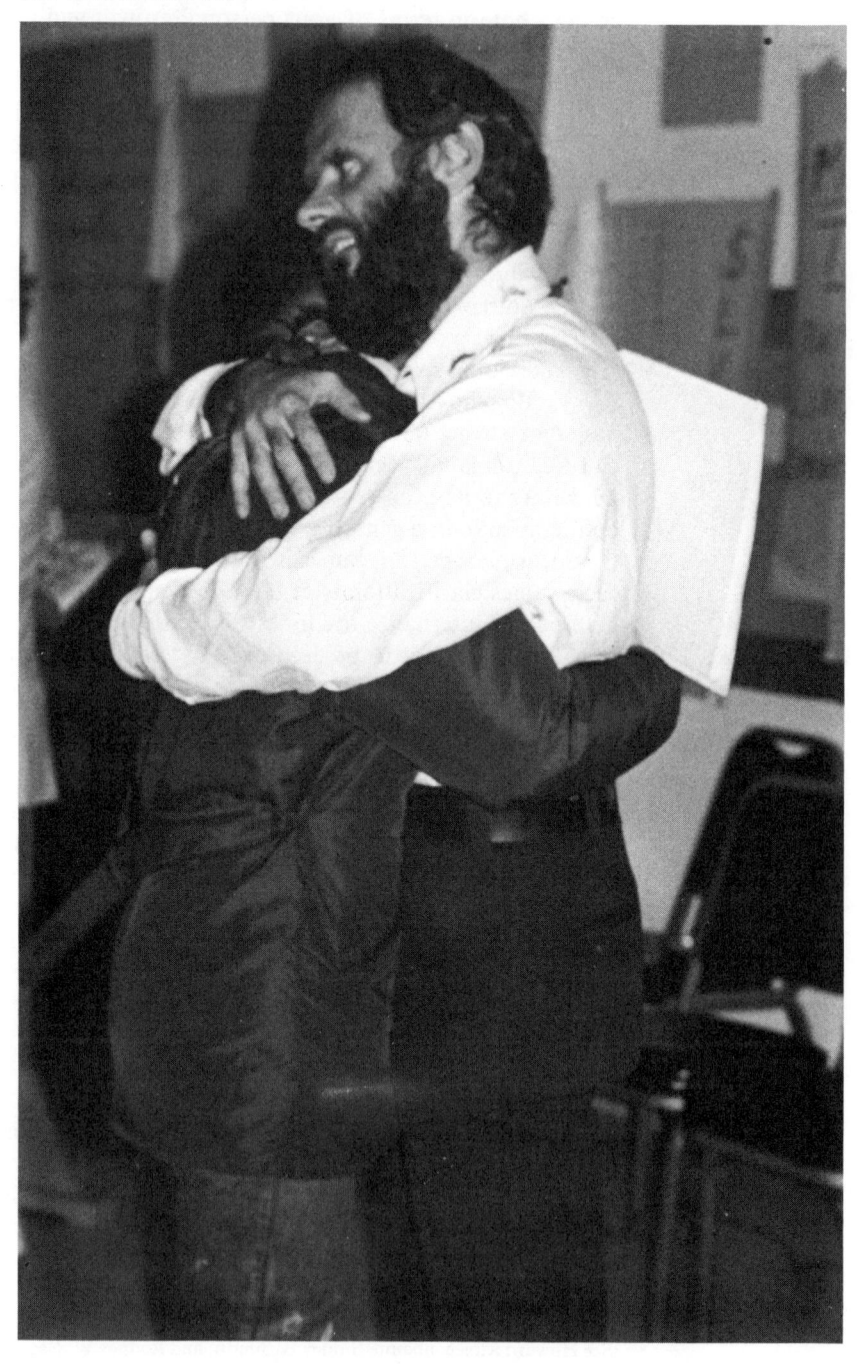

18 Stay awake to the danger of the "One Hundred Things I Love to Do" syndrome. This often occurs when more than one teacher in the building is involved with values clarification. What happens is that during the first period, students in English class do the inventory "Twenty Things I Love to Do in Life." When second period rolls around, the social-studies teacher hits them with the same inventory. And so on through the five periods of the school day. It is vital for teachers to talk with one another (intra- as well as interdepartmentally) and to develop short-range and long-range goals for integrating values clarification in the classroom.

19 In relation to this, it is vitally important that the teacher be sensitive to the needs and *readiness* of the students. What may "work" in one class might fall flat in another. Stay tuned in to your students.

20 Seek support from colleagues and friends. Many people realize the value of support and have moved on to formalizing support systems for themselves. For example, the National Humanistic Education Center (110 Spring Street, Saratoga Springs, New York 12866) is encouraging people to form local support groups that might engage in any of the following: sharing values-clarification strategies, brainstorming new strategies, discussing readings, problem-solving, developing facilitating skills, creating values units in curricula, learning about the "cousins" of values clarification (related fields in humanistic education).

SUMMARY

We are concerned—both ethically and strategically—with how values clarification is used. We are concerned about people who find themselves in the same kind of swamp as the toad we met at the beginning of the chapter. And we want to respond to people who want to know, "What's the score?" when it comes to implementing values clarification.

In this chapter, we have offered a score of ideas that you can use in leapfrogging off this book. We have included them with an attitude of caring (for you, the reader, and for your students), and not with an attitude of "We toad [sic] you so."

APPENDICES

TERMINOLOGY

What is nice about any new movement is that it often brings with it a whole new vocabulary. This is no less true of humanistic education. Terms like "alone time," "focusing," and "here and now" are used and referred to as common expressions of how to do it and what is being done. They also help in gaining a greater understanding of and appreciation for the whole process of humanistic education.

Here we provide you with some of the terms that we use in working with values in the classroom and in workshops. We think they will strengthen your understanding of and ability to work with values in your own unique situation.

Active listening (focusing)

This is one aspect of communication that encourages the individual or group to listen (to focus) in on that person who has the floor. When one person is talking, the others may *not* contribute any statements and may only ask questions that will truly help to clarify what the individual is trying to say. The concept of active listening helps to train individuals to really listen to what is being said, rather than to be half-listening, and/or half-rehearsing, or thinking about, what they will say in reply.

Affective education

The complement of cognitive education (that of dealing with facts only) in that one deals with feelings, values, etc.

Alone time

This is private, unstructured time in which the student can think, write, and reflect. It is suggested that at least five minutes be provided during the last session of the week for this kind of private consideration of the experiences, activities, and learnings that the classes are providing. Students may be encouraged to add personal statements to their journals, or write a brief letter to the teacher expressing certain feelings. The important element is that although the teacher may make some suggestions, this time is for the student to do with as she/he wishes.

Brainstorming

This is a technique for generating ideas quickly with a group of people (or by yourself). It can be both fun and creative, and can produce many ideas within a short period. Some of the guidelines for effective brainstorming include:

people in the group call out ideas while one or two others record ideas;

no discussion of a single idea is allowed during the brainstorming session;

no evaluative remarks are permitted, positive or negative, as this inhibits the free flow of ideas;

the group is encouraged to build (piggyback) on each other's statements;

allow all ideas to be recorded, however "ridiculous" they may seem; and,

limit the brainstorming session to three to six minutes; never let it drag on.

Closure

At this point, most often at the end of an exercise and/or discussion, participants are asked to make some final, individual comment(s) about the learning activity. The focus should be on either their personal reactions to the experience, or the ways in which they did or did not benefit from the experience.

APPENDICES

Facilitator

The teacher relinquishes his/her role as authority figure and begins to assume the role of facilitator (Postman and Weingartner, 1973). Rather than "teaching" per se, the teacher guides the student through a problem, using a technique that is nonjudgmental and accepting. The goal is to help the individual to come to his or her own conclusions.

Fantasy

Daydreaming is a universal experience. For the normal, well-adjusted person, it is a wholesome form of relaxation, a "getting-away-from-it-all." This fantasy world can be tapped as a source of information in the classroom as well as a source of power for the individual. Whether watching a film, thinking, writing, we often ask the students to share their fantasies. Such sharing can often reveal more about a person than "reality" thinking.

Feedback

As individuals learn to work together, they discover many ways of checking with each other (getting feedback), so that distortions are reduced. As one student expresses a feeling, others in the group may be asked to give this person feedback on what they "heard the person say," what they "feel about what was said," is what was said "consistent with what this person has said and done in the past?" and the like. In another sense, feedback may be used throughout the entire process, whereby participants should feel free at all times to make any comments concerning the process employed and/or the methods being used by the group, teacher.

I learned (relearned) statements

This is a form of statement that can be used by the teacher at any time. The general format is for the teacher to ask the students to respond to the statement "I learned . . ." Any experiential verb may be used, depending on the situation. Some other examples include: "I relearned that I . . .," "I discovered . . .," "I realized . . .," "I felt [or feel] . . . ." The purpose of such statements is to give the students an opportunity to explore their feelings, based on certain experiences that they have encountered in the class or workshop. For example, after the students watch a particular film, you might ask them to write two or more "I learned [or relearned] . . ." statements.

Inventory

An inventory is the listing and examination of specific behavior or patterns within very specific limits. It is an important basic tool in helping one learn more about oneself. An example of a simple inventory would be to ask students to list five of the most satisfying learning experiences they have had in the past week.

Killer statements

Killer statements or put-downs are one of the best ways of cutting off creative thinking and sharing in a classroom. Using this technique is also one of the best ways of preventing others from sharing, or worse, causing them to become hostile or defensive. Killer statements include: "You can't be serious?" "That was a dumb statement!" "How could you say such a thing!" "I would never look at it that way!" Being aware of killer statements and put-downs is the first step in improving communication in the classroom and freeing students to be able to be more authentic. How do you foster an atmosphere that is free of killer statements? By discussion and explanation, by brainstorming all the possible verbal put-downs (and the nonverbal ones as well), by role-playing situations where one person is trying to put another down, or by asking students to keep a record of all the put-downs that they hear in the course of the day. Even more important is showing students ways in which to channel their energy toward finding or seeking out the positive and worth in each individual. It would also be helpful to point out to students the fact that killer statements represent one of the life positions described by Dr. Eric Berne, namely "I'm OK—You're not OK". (Berne, 1964.)

Negotiating

To negotiate is to attempt to work out certain differences with another person or to arrive at a mutual agreement on a particular matter. If two students or student and "teacher" disagree on a particular matter, we sometimes ask them to attempt to negotiate, to work out a formula that is mutually agreed on by both parties.

Peer-group pressure

In any group there is always present the aspect of peer pressure and controls that affect the feelings, thoughts, and behavior of individual group members. The teacher should be aware that these are powerful influences, especially with the young, and should therefore learn to read and work with these pressures. The teacher may even find it worthwhile to spend some time working with one or two value exercises that deal with group pressure.

Positive focus

It seems that the system has for years been concerned primarily with providing students with negative focuses. Grades, marking off for spelling, and marking off for late papers are among these negatives. The concept of positive focus (as is true of positive "strokes") is based on the principle that the teacher and the class begin to focus on the positive aspects of each individual. Look for the good in each thought, each feeling and point, each word that is shared, and point this positive aspect out to the individual and the class. With practice, students will begin to find it easier and easier to consider the positive worth in each individual rather than the negative.

Positive "strokes"

It seems that we spend a great deal of our time telling people about all the negative or bad things that we recognize or see in them. The concept of positive "strokes" means that we begin to recognize the positive aspects of an individual and share these positive feelings with them. A simple positive "stroke" exercise is to mark all the right answers on a student's paper rather than using an X to mark all the wrong answers.

Processing

Processing is an essential and most important part of EVERY exercise. In fact, it is what makes an exercise or activity either worthwhile or worthless. Processing falls into two general types:
1 *From the teacher.* Examples here may include:

allowing an opportunity for review of what has happened during the activity;

trying to identify certain feelings that occur during an activity or at different points during the activity;

trying to point out and identify different behaviors, thoughts, feelings in an activity;

noting behavioral changes that take place during or after an activity or experience;

pointing out the need to try on new patterns of acting and behaving;

identifying and giving recognition to any unfinished business generated by the activity.

In short, at the end of an exercise the teacher's role is that of providing feedback, asking provocative questions, and pointing out obvious (and not so obvious) patterns of behavior.

2 *From the student.* The student should be able to provide herself or himself with feedback on what has occurred. By this we mean that not only does she/he go through the exercise, but that they begin to understand the reasons underlying his or her feelings, attitudes, and behavior. The teacher can help the student to analyze his or her own behavior, a process we call self-evaluation. This knowledge can be utilized in his or her own positive self-growth. The types of questions that are often found to be most valuable here are:

Did you note any differences between your behavior and the behavior of others?

What prevented you from acting in a different way than you did? Or, did not allow you to do so?

Do you see a pattern in your responses?

How would you fantasize your parents' response if they were given this situation?

Can you fantasize what would happen to you if you had responded differently?

Risk-taking

This is a most important concept, for it is very much related to personal growth. By risk-taking we mean the chance one often takes when one ventures out of one's pattern of behavior. The risk is in having one's feelings hurt, of being rejected, belittled, or in other ways offended. But the risk is often worth the potential pain, for if a person can be open and free even with only one other person, there is a greater likelihood that one can be in touch with oneself. It is safe to say that regardless of the risk involved, the greatest risk would come from not exercising the opportunity to risk—and possibly grow from it. Some encouraging words that the teacher can offer to a student who is hesitant are: "What is the worst thing that could happen to you if you did risk?" "If you do not risk where will you be?" "Is the potential for positive gain greater than the risk?"

Role-playing

Role-playing is a method for studying the attitudes and feelings of individuals in simulated situations. Group members are asked to take different roles, and improvise dialogue and action to fit the role or problem situation. In this kind of situation group members may learn more about their own attitudes and behavior and try to find new ways of dealing with their problems. Role-playing is usually followed by a free discussion of what went on and how the actors and observers (if any) felt about the interactions. Role-playing is a form of psychodrama. (Moreno, 1946.)

Self-concept

A person's self-concept comprises all his/her beliefs about who he/she is. It includes one's assumptions about one's strength and weakness, one's possibilities for growth, and it includes one's explicit descriptions of one's customary patterns of behavior and experiencing. If you were asked to describe yourself you would give a picture of who and what you are (your self-concept). Yet, one's self-concept is not so much descriptive of experience and action as it is prescriptive. The self-concept is a commitment. (Jourard, 1974.)

Self-disclosure

What we reveal is pretty much up to us, although not entirely so. Sometimes pressure from conflicting forces opens doors for accidental disclosure. In group work, one is often asked or forced to disclose oneself. Certainly self-disclosure can lead to growth, but as Sidney Jourard has stated, transparency is not necessarily a mark of soundness in a person, nor an indication of depth in a relationship. The key is in the appropriateness in self-disclosure, the balance of spontaneity and discretion reflecting the nature of the relationship. (Jourard, 1974.)

Self-evaluation

By self-evaluation we mean that people really begin to evaluate their own behavior, really look at themselves. Values clarification is a useful technique for helping people to look at themselves in terms of what they are doing and how they are behaving, and to try and identify certain patterns they feel are productive or unproductive.

Sharing

In group work, one is often asked to share. By this we mean that the individual is asked to talk to others about his or her feelings and thoughts, concerning an experience that has taken place, a reaction to an exercise, or feelings about another.

Significant others

These are people who usually would not necessarily be identified as friends but who *are important* to the individual for a variety of reasons. A teacher who has had a real impact on a student, a particularly successful athlete, or a student leader whom one may admire, or even a neighborhood bully—all these people may be significant or important in the development of the individual.

Strategy

A strategy is simply an exercise or an activity that helps give the student a better understanding of a particular concern or conflict she or he may be working through. It may also bring into focus new ways of viewing certain things. The exercises are structured carefully to help students deal with personal areas in such a way that they will begin to learn more about themselves. The exercises always observe the basic rules and are always processed in some way.

Support groups

Support groups are made up of those people (usually six to eight in number) who would like to work together; feel a desire to "support" each other even though they may not always agree; desire to work together for a certain period of time; and, develop a certain degree of trust with each other and thus feel more free to share their true feelings. In a large group (twenty-five or more) we often find it more productive to have group members develop support groups (usually through some form of self-selection), and to stay with their support group. In this way it is easy to have a large group go through an exercise and then say, "Now get into your support groups and share feelings about that exercise!" or to have them get into their support groups and then go through an exercise and share feelings. At the end of the day or class we unite the whole group again.

Taking Responsibility for oneself

We almost always say in a workshop or class, "Take responsibility for yourself!" It goes without saying that when someone feels unable or is afraid to express his or her authentic feelings about certain issues that may be raised, then the goal of self affirmation, discovery, and expression will be blocked in some way. That occurs because there is a considerable amount of "risk-taking" that becomes an integral part of the class. It is quite different, for example, for a student to say, "I personally feel that the research available does not prove that homosexuality is a sickness!" and "I am a homosexual, and I do not feel that I am sick!" Ways of helping students to begin to take responsibility for themselves include:

When speaking, try saying, "I feel . . ."
Try saying, "I won't . . ." instead of, "I can't . . ."
Try saying, "I heard you say . . ." instead of, "You said . . ."
Always speak in the first person.
Remember that you, as facilitator, must also adhere to these important rules.

Teacher-modeling

The teacher is an extremely important role model in the class. Therefore, it is important that the teacher be a positive model in terms of openness; able to share feelings; and capable of active listening and accepting others' values, feelings, and different points of view. In short, don't expect your students to share if you don't expect yourself to share.

Trust

Trust is an important ingredient in the humanistic process. This trust has three major elements: (1) that each student trust himself—what he or she feels, what she/he values, and how she/he responds in various situations. In short, that she/he not feel constrained or threatened by self or others; (2) that each person develop this same degree of trust in others that she/he has developed in the self; and, (3) that the teacher share in this trusting—that she/he trusts and is trusted.

REFERENCES

Bach, George, and Deutsch, Ronald M. *Pairing.* New York: Avon Books, 1970

Berne, Eric, *Games People Play.* New York: Grove Press, 1964.

Brown, George Isaac. *Human Teaching for Human Learning.* New York: Viking Press, 1971.

Glasser, William. *Schools Without Failure.* New York: Harper & Row, 1969.

Greer, Mary, and Rubinstein, Bonnie. *Will the Real Teacher Please Stand Up: A Primer in Humanistic Education.* Pacific Palisades, Calif.: Goodyear Publishing Co., 1972.

Hawley, Robert C. *Human Values in the Classroom.* Amherst, Mass.: Education Research Associates, 1973.

Jourard, Sidney M. *Healthy Personality.* New York: Macmillan Publishing Co., 1974.

Luft, Joseph. *Of Human Interaction.* Palo Alto, Calif.: National Press Books, 1969.

Moreno, J. L. *Psychodrama.* New York: Beacon House, 1946.

Overly, Norman V., ed. *The Unstudied Curriculum: Its Impact on Children.* Washington, D.C.: Association for Supervision and Curriculum Development, 1970.

Perls, Frederick S. *Gestalt Therapy Verbatim.* Lafayette, Calif.: Real People Press, 1969.

Postman, Neil, and Weingartner, Charles. *The School Book.* New York: Delacorte Press, 1969.

156 APPENDICES

Prince, George M. *The Practice of Creativity: A Manual for Dynamic Group Problem Solving.* New York: Harper & Row, 1970.

Raths, Louis E.; Harmin, Merrill; and Simon, Sidney B. *Values and Teaching: Working With Values in the Classroom.* Columbus, Ohio: Charles E. Merrill Publishing Co., 1966.

Rubin, Louis. "Curriculum, Affect, and Humanism," *Educational Leadership* (October 1974): 10–13.

Shaftel, Fannie R., and Shaftel, George. *Role-playing for Social Values: Decision-Making in the Social Studies.* Englewood Cliffs, N.J.: Prentice-Hall, Inc., 1967.

Simon, Sidney B.; Hartwell, Marie R.; and Hawkins, Laurance A. "Values Clarification: Friends & Other People," unpublished, 1973.

Weinstein, Gerald, and Fantini, Mario D., eds. *Toward Humanistic Education: A Curriculum of Affect.* New York: Praeger Publishers, 1970.

_____, and Alschuler, Alfred. "Developmental Self-Knowledge: A Humanistic Education Goal," Amherst, Mass.: University of Massachusetts, School of Education, Working Paper #1, August, 1973.

ADDITIONAL VALUES SHEETS: A SAMPLING

Sexuality[1]

No matter how sensual you are, there will be days when you don't feel like making love. You may have a cold, or be extremely tired from overwork and pressure or, somehow, no matter how you push it and will it, have trouble getting your body to come completely alive. That happens to all women, even sexy you.

But men's sexual drives don't always coincide with women's peaks. Quite often men are most ardent during female lows.

There are times when you can quite legitimately say, "I love you, but I can't make love right now," but no woman of any sensitivity would refuse to make love to a man she cares for, just because she "doesn't really feel like it." You focus like mad on all the fantasies that stir your sexual juices, concentrate on making your body respond to the highest point possible and, if you really can't get to orgasm, to avoid disappointing him and spoiling his plateau of excitement and sexiness, you fake that orgasm.[2]

To Think and Write about

1 *Write your reaction to the quotation above in just a few words.*

---

[1] Thanks to David M. Goodman for sharing this values sheet with us.

[2] "J." THE SENSUOUS WOMAN. © 1969 by Lyle Stuart Inc. Published by arrangement with Lyle Stuart, Inc.

157 APPENDICES

2 *Under what circumstances would you "fake it?"*

3 *What do you feel are the possible consequences of "faking it" in a relationship?"*

4 *How would you feel if you discovered your partner had "faked it?"*

5 *What do you think are possible alternatives to "faking it" in a relationship?*

Some other things to chew on

1 Beyond the sexual aspect of a relationship, in what other areas would you expect to find people "faking it?"
2 In your relationships with other people, when are you most likely to "fake it?"
3 Is your response to the last question consistent with the response you made to question 2 in the previous section just above?

"Loving means touching"[3]

In the ruthless world of business, we can dismiss a girl with whom we have only shaken hands, or we can betray a colleague with whom we have only shaken hands, or we can betray a colleague with whom we have done no more than rest a hand on a shoulder; but what if the body contacts had been greater? What if, without any sexual involvement, we had experienced greater intimacies with them? Then, without a doubt, we would have seen our tough determination soften, and our competitiveness dwindle, when the moments for brutal decisions came. And if we dare not expose ourselves to these dangers, to these powerful reciprocal involvements that know no logic, then we certainly do not want to be reminded of them by seeing them flaunted in public by others. So the young lovers can keep to themselves and do it in private, and in case they ignore our request we will make it law. We will make it a crime to be intimate in public. And so it is that, even to this day, in certain sophisticated, civilized countries it remains a crime to kiss in public. A tender act of touching becomes immoral and illegal. A gentle intimacy becomes legally equated with an act of theft. So hide it away quickly, lest the rest of us see what we are missing![4]

[3]Thanks to Bruce G. Mitchell for sharing this one with us.
[4]Desmond Morris. INTIMATE BEHAVIOUR. New York: Random House, 1972, p. 151.

158 APPENDICES

1 *Write your reactions to the paragraph above, Do it quickly. Don't even write full sentences.*

2 *What implications does the view presented here have for your own life?*

3 *Can you list some things you did in the past that might well have broken your relationships with other people?*

4 *What can you do to change your own life by becoming more intimate with others?*

Homosexuality[5]   Picture, if you will, an apartment building containing, of course, people. In apartment 4E live two young women. Below, in apartment 3E, a man lives alone. From what may be assumed as "reliable sources," the man in 3E discovers that the two women above are lesbians. Mr. "3E" has never met the Misses "4E" and has never been bothered (from 4E) by the more common types of apartment harassment (e.g. such as loud parties, foot tapping). From the moment the man learned the women were gay, he experienced great anxiety and was unable to sleep at night. So, he went about doing all he could think of to get the lesbians evicted.

You are a fly on a dormitory wall. You've been observing Douglas and Charles for some time. They seem to be very comfortable with one another, in that they are easily able to embrace one another out of the joy of really liking, understanding, and empathizing with one another. In fact, you see that they are able to be entirely intimate with one another. On this particular occasion, you are perched high on the corridor wall just opposite Doug and Chuck's door, which happens to be open. They appear to be very intimate right now. Down the hall comes a group of people who take note of and stop outside the open door. At first you hear constrained giggling, which soon breaks into open laughter and eventually becomes loud cries of "FAIRIES, QUEERS, FAGGOTS!"

1 *Without commenting on the likelihood of these two stories, write your reactions to them. Do it quickly. Don't write full sentences.*

[5]Thanks to Leonard B. Chandler, III, for sharing this one with us.

2 *Do you know any gay people? How did you react to the discovery they were gay? How do you react to them now?*

3 *Would you react differently if you discovered that a close relative (e.g. daughter/son, sister/brother, mother/father) were gay? Why or why not?*

Apartment four upstairs

Today I wondered about love
   And saw an old couple returning from the market,
  She with her varicose legs
     Like splotches of grape jelly on bread,
  He with his swollen, arthritic knee
     And emphysema wheeze.
They paused at the bottom of shaky, white steps
And grinned when he handed her the grocery bag.
  She went first, painfully, slowly,
   He followed, stiff hands pushing her rump.
And at the top he gently goosed her.
  She shrieked a bit, he coughed,
They laughed and disappeared inside apartment four upstairs.[6]

1 *What do you like best about this old couple?*

2 *Someday you'll be old; what will you miss most?*

3 *What are some things you can do now to assure that you'll have spirit then?*

4 *Whom have you goosed or been goosed by lately, and what does it mean?*

5 *Have you any further comments on this value sheet?*

[6]James Kavanaugh.

Parenting

Linda Pratt failed to return home from a dance Friday night. On Saturday she admitted she had spent the night with an Air Force Lieutenant. The Pratts decided on a punishment that would "wake Linda up." They ordered her to shoot the dog she had owned about two years. On Sunday, the Pratts and Linda took the dog into the desert near their home. They had the girl dig a shallow grave. Then Ms. Pratt grasped the dog between her hand and Mr. Pratt gave his daughter a .22 caliber pistol and told her to shoot the dog. Instead, the girl put the pistol to her right temple and shot herself. The police said there were no charges that could be filed against the parents except possibly cruelty to animals.[7]

Would You Share Some Feelings?

1 *Write down your first reaction to what you have just read:*

2 *Who do you feel was (were) the most violent person(s) in this story?*
   a Linda, who may have slept with the lieutenant?
   b the Air Force Lieutenant who took advantage of Linda?
   c Mr. and Ms. Pratt, who ordered the dog shot?
   d The police, who could find no charges to be filed?
   e The society that permitted this to happen and offered no corrective action?

3 *What implications does this story have for your life?*

4 *What alternative actions could you have suggested (if any) for Linda's parents?*

5 *What would you have felt if you were the daughter of Mr. and Ms. Pratt?*

Love and sex[8]

Women play at sex in order to get love: Men play at love in order to get sex.[9]

[7] The *New York Times* Company, 1968.

[8] Thanks to David M. Goodman for sharing this one with us.

[9] Article in the *Daily Free Press*.

To think and write about:

1. Do you identify with the quote above? In what way?

2. Where do your current attitudes, beliefs, and feelings about sex come from?

3. How is your behavior in the areas of love and sex consistent with your attitudes, beliefs, and feelings?

4. What are the possible ways of handling a situation in which you felt you were being manipulated by a member of the opposite sex?

5. If the quotation above suggests a problem that worries you, are there some things you might personally do about it? Within yourself? Within the larger society?

Why we smoke

Early warnings of damage from cigarette smoking are so subtle as to be almost entirely missed or ignored by persons involved. . . . They put up with a chronic cough, and a drizzly nose-and-throat, and a gravel voice, and a bird cage mouth. The gradual increase in cough and spitting, the slow decline in wind and a little bit duller feeling in the head from day to day are met with genial equanimity until the growing cancer, failing heart, and destruction of lung tissue are all too solid an established fact. . . . "I'll smoke until I get into trouble and then I'll quit, and be okay." This is truly a fool's solution since the worst harm from smoking gives no alarm until it is far too late to make a recovery—this is the secret of the danger. . . . The smoker who waits for an unmistakable warning has, for the most part, waited too long. . . .

And why is extra pressure put on you to start smoking by advertising? To put it in the cruelest possible way, each of you, like a slave on the block many years ago, is worth up to a cool $8,000—the amount that the privilege of smoking will cost you in a lifetime, provided you live to a reasonable age. You are worth that if you get started—hooked solid between now and the time you are 20 and to do this the advertising bends every effort.

Tobacco today brings in about $8 billion a year and you are expected to pay your dues to the smoker's club which, interestingly and significantly, runs to about the same amount as does the national bill for all doctors' services. To get you contributing in good style, the best in the U.S. advertising skills are concentrated on you; and to succeed they use an interesting theme.

The gimmick? You guessed it. Smoking makes you manly, not old-manly: fliers, cowboys, hunters, professional athletes, young executives, great lovers and even beautiful girls. But you seldom if ever see a brand advertised by showing grandma or grandpa lighting up, because the emphasis is on you, not grandpa or even dad. They are hooked now (or never will start). The bait is for you.

May I remind you again that the quota in young people—in you—is 4,500 of you fresh, new "fish" each day, even though the packages now must show that "smoking may be dangerous to health," in clear print. This little sign doesn't say how, or when or how much—and it never will and I might add that by law no further truth can be added until 1972; this sign can't be changed until then.

The worst part of it all is that you not only pay for the cigarettes, to be mature and glamorous, but you also pay for entrapping advertising. Socrates had nothing on you when he had to pay for the poison. Indeed, you pay the whole thing if you let them make a sucker out of you and the final statement on your bill reads: "Debit: Your health and perhaps your life."[10]

To think and write about:

1 *Write your reaction to this statement on smoking.*

2 *Can you remember, if you are a smoker, when, how, and why you got started smoking?*

How can you keep your children from starting?

3 *Can you, as an individual, do anything about this problem? If not you, who can do something about it?*

How do you process research information?

Grass linked to fertility loss

BOSTON (AP)—Men who smoke large amounts of marijuana run risks of decreased production of male sex hormones and sperm which could affect their fertility, researchers say.

In tests with 20 heavy marijuana users who smoked from five to 18 "joints" a week for months or longer, researchers found that 35 per cent had noticeably decreased sperm counts. They also found that blood levels of the hormone testosterone averaged 44 per cent lower in the drug users than nonusers.

[10]Excerpts from a talk to students, Phillips Academy, Andover, Mass., by Frank P. Foster, M.D., Assistant Clinical Professor of Medicine, Boston University, 1971.

In a report published yesterday in the New England Journal of Medicine, the researchers said two of the chronic smokers were impotent "apparently in association with marijuana use."

The report noted that one of these men returned to normal sexuality within two months after he discontinued marijuana use, but the other declined to give up the drug.

The study was conducted at the Reproductive Biology Research Foundation in St. Louis, and its director, noted sex researcher Dr. William H. Masters was one of the report's authors. Others conducting the study were Drs. Robert Kolodny and Gelson Toro, and Robert M. Kolodner.

The study noted that the results should be taken cautiously because of the small size of the sample, lack of data on the potency of the marijuana and because it was impossible to measure hormone levels and sperm counts of the marijuana users before they took up the drug.

The researchers said their examinations of the 18 to 28-year-old users, who were compared with 20 similarly healthy men of the same age who did not use the drug, showed no noticeable change in testicular size or texture in the users.

The study said the depressant effects of heavy marijuana use on both sperm count and testosterone levels seemed directly related to the amount of marijuana used. Subjects averaging more than 10 marijuana cigarettes weekly had significantly lower testosterone than less chronic users, the researchers said.

The male hormone finding is of particular significance, the researchers said, because numerous other research findings indicate that a lack of testosterone at critical points in the development of a male fetus can cause sex organs to develop improperly and later cause permanent hormone imbalance in the male offspring.

The researchers said it would be "judicious" for women to avoid marijuana at least during the first three months of pregnancy since it has been shown that marijuana ingredients can pass from the mother to the fetus.

The study hypothesized that a pre-adolescent boy who was a heavy marijuana smoker possibly could throw off his puberty since this depends on proper hormone balance.

Looking at the often-voiced boasts of marijuana and performance, the researchers remarked that the assertions probably should be reassessed.

Questions to think and write about:

1 *Does this research impress you? Comment.*

2 *How would you approach a heavy marijuana user if you were worried about his ruining his fertility?*

3 *Can you cite some research that impressed you enough to change your habits, patterns, or even your life?*

4 *What else do you want to say that has been motivated by this sheet?*

Smoking

Recent tests show that the average smoker spends only 20 seconds actually inhaling his cigarette. During the 10 to 12 minutes of burning, its output of tar and nicotine is up to four times greater than during the time that it is actually being puffed. Thus, a non-smoker in a smoke-filled room may actually be forced against his will to breathe almost as much cigarette smoke as the actual smoker sitting next to him. Is that fair? The speaker, John Banzhaf III, a Washington, D.C., attorney and executive director of Action on Smoking and Health (ASH), thinks that it is not. And his organization is attempting to do something about it. "Unrestricted smoking, even in confined public places, is nothing short of a national disgrace," he adds. "For far too long we have been the silent majority, afraid to speak up when someone polluted our lungs." Interested individuals can contact ASH at 2000 H. St., N.W., Washington, D.C. 20006.[11]

Questions to think and write about:

1 *Are you in basic agreement or disagreement with Mr. Banzhaf? Explain.*

2 *Some people have put up no-smoking signs in their homes and cars. Does that seem like an imposition to you? Explain.*

3 *Where do you stand on the idea that all smokers should ask, "Do you mind if I smoke?" before they light up, and if someone says, "No," they should smoke, but if someone says, "I do mind . . ." they should not smoke?*

4 *If you are a nonsmoker, what would you be willing to give up that is as hard for a smoker to give up? Why don't you?*

5 *List five things you would like to live by in terms of the entire issue raised by this values sheet?*

[11]Eco Notes: *Northwest Passage;* 8–21 November 1971.

What's your opinion?

Read the statement below and comment on it:

"I never have, and never will eat any animal foods. They are unhealthy. I won't allow my children to eat them either."

1 *What's your first reaction to the above statement?*

2 *Do you think of the statement as being a healthy or unhealthy one?*

3 *Do you, or could you, live by the attitude proposed in the statement? Why, or why not?*

4 *If you disagree with the statement, list three different ways to modify its meaning so as to better reflect your own values.*

Insights

The rising price of sugar has set me thinking about why sugar is so appealing to so many.

It is reported that as a country becomes more prosperous, the demand for sugar increases. This may indicate that as economic security is assured a desire for pleasurable experiences becomes more pronounced. It seems to me that eating sweets is one way of filling this need, but I wonder if the craving for sweet tasting foods may not really be a craving for sweet sensations of any sort. Then because it may be easier to taste something sweet than it is to call upon our other senses to enjoy the sweet things of life, we may tend to focus on this one area.

Perhaps we should use this sweet-food craving as just an indication of the real desire and rely on other senses to satisfy it as, for example, by listening to beautiful music or by viewing beauty in nature or art. All our senses are capable of perceiving sweetness. Why rely on taste alone?[12]

Questions to think and write about:

1 *What is your reaction to the writer's argument?*

---

[12]Molly Berotti, in *The Bucks County R.C. Newsletter*.

2   What is your pattern of eating sweets? What eating binges do you go on? What sweet things draw you when you are feeling less good about yourself?

3   Make a list of other "sweet" experiences that you have enjoyed and might well enjoy instead of reaching for a sugar sweet.

4   Are you serious about changing your life in this way? Where do you begin? What help do you need from us?

FILMS IN VALUES CLARIFICATION

The films here can be used as motivational films, training in the area of values clarification, or as sources of data to work with in terms of issues that can spark discussion and questioning.

A Strategy for Teaching Values. Guidance Associates. (10 min.; 10 min.; 6 min. three filmstrips; two cassettes). Includes theoretical background on values clarification, examples of implementation, and a discussion model for children.

Clarifying Your Values: Guidelines for Living. The Center for Humanities, Inc. (two carousels; a hundred sixty slides with tape cassettes; color). The program encourages students to define their value systems by analyzing their day-to-day reactions to people and events.

Conflict in American Values: Life Style vs Standard of Living. The Center for Humanities, Inc. (two carousels; one hundred sixty slides with tape cassettes; color). Investigates evolving American values, giving particular attention to the current debate over pursuit of special life styles rather than the attainment of a certain standard of living.

Exploring Moral Values by Louis E. Raths. Warren Schloat Productions, Inc. (filmstrips). Fifteen individual filmstrips dealing with questions about alternatives in life situations. Issues dealt with are prejudice, personal values, authority, honesty.

Future Shock. McGraw-Hill (42 min.; color). This dramatic documentary, based on the Alvin Toffler best seller, explores the impact of exponentially accelerating change in individuals, institutions and their values.

Hard Choices: Strategies for Decision Making. The Center for Humanities, Inc. (two carousels; one hundred sixty slides with tape cassettes; color). This program is structured to teach students a series of decision-making skills and help them evaluate the risks involved in making decisions about real life situations such as marriage.

Replay. McGraw-Hill (8 min.; color). Is today that different from yesterday, or do we merely think it is? As middle-aged interviewees criticize the "youth culture," fast cuts to scenes of their "good old days" reveal an amazing continuity.

String Bean. McGraw-Hill (17 min.; black and white). An old woman plants a seed from a string bean, but the plant soon grows too large for her tiny flat, so she transfers it to the public garden. Later, the gardeners discover the alien growth and destroy it. Undaunted, the woman takes a bean from her dead plant and begins to grow a new one.

That's Me. McGraw-Hill (15 min.; color). A social worker attempts to "redeem" a young Puerto Rican who would rather play his guitar in Central Park than go to school or work. In the end, the roles reverse. It is the social worker who cannot function within the system he has chosen. *That's Me* questions acceptance of a traditional system that does not always fit the individual, and examines priorities for personal fulfillment.

The Adolescent Experience: Developing Values. Guidance Associates (7 and 10 minutes. two filmstrips; two cassettes). Part I dramatizes a developmental sequence of values-forming episodes: parental punishment-reward experiences, peer influences. In part II, students are required to make value choices after watching three open-ended vignettes.

The Ialac Story, Fuzzies, and *Why Am I Afraid To Tell You Who I Am?* Argus Communications (filmstrips 8 to 27 min.). Animated filmstrips dealing with feelings of hurt, rejection, joy, sharing, and role-playing.

Time Piece. McGraw-Hill (10 min.; color). From the confines of his hospital bed, one man relives the nightmare fantasy of the dehumanizing race with death that is his life. In rejecting the destructive values and goals of a frenzied civilization, the film demands a search for values to counter the effects of a dehumanizing society.

Toys. McGraw-Hill (8 min.; color). As a group of enthralled children watch, the war toys in a shop window come to life and enact the real-life horrors they represent. The children remain frozen in terror, even after the toys return to normal. How do seemingly insignificant objects shape our values? How does society perpetuate its values?

Values Clarification Program. Sunburst Communications (filmstrips). Four extremely interesting and provocative open-ended stories for teaching values and the concepts of discrimination and prejudice.

Values for Dating. Sunburst Communications (filmstrips). Investigates the attitudes of young people regarding two important dating areas: love and sex.

Values for Teenagers in the 1970s. Guidance Associates (9 and 11 min.; two filmstrips; two cassettes). Part I focuses on specific problems often central to social and personal decision-making: sex, drinking, cigarette smoking. Part II examines the dynamics of peer-group pressure, acceptance, conformity.

Vignette Films. Paulist Productions (12 min.; color). A series of 11 films each lasting 12 minutes. Each film challenges the students to clarify their values, explore alternatives, and accelerate the process of their own personal growth. Film titles are:
Close Feelings
Different with Dignity
Rapport
Walls and Windows
Kinships
Me, Myself
Being Real
The Price of Life
Daily Bread
Priorities
A Place to Stand

Wall. McGraw-Hill (4 min.; color). Two men approach an impassable wall. One sits down to wait. The other attempts to overcome the obstacle in a number of inventive ways, failing each time. Finally, in frustration, he batters his head through the wall, killing himself. The other man steps through the wall, comes to another, and sits down to wait. The film explores conflicting value systems in a problem-solving context. The different levels of meaning depend on our interpretation of the wall.

Film sources

Argus Communications
7440 Natchez Avenue
Niles, Ill. 60648

Guidance Associates
757 Third Avenue
New York, New York 10017

McGraw-Hill Book Co., Inc.
330 West 42nd Street
New York, New York 10036

Paulist Productions
P.O. Box 1057
Pacific Palisades, Calif. 90272

Sunburst Communications
39 Washington Avenue
Pleasantville, New York 10570

The Center for Humanities, Inc.
2 Holland Avenue
White Plains, New York 10603

Warren Schloat Productions, Inc.
Pleasantville, New York 10570

TAPES AND CASSETTES IN VALUES CLARIFICATION

Making Sense of Our Lives by Merrill Harmin. Each side of a cassette tape contains a complete group activity: a dramatization in story, music, and narration. Suggested questions and activities follow the dramatizations and are included on the sound track. Each activity is coordinated with a spirit master you can use to expand the ideas and questions introduced on the sound track.

Cassette I

Side 1: *The Problem of Hunger.* Students are challenged with the question of when, if ever, a person who is desperate for food may justifiably steal.
Side 2: *The Gift of Idealism.* A folk ballad introduces questions about idealism and self-sacrifice.

Cassette II

Side 1: *Personal Reetionships.* A look at the meaning of friendship and communication between friends.
Side 2: *Dear Merrill.* The narrator asks everyone to try writing a letter, real or imaginary, about a problem, and, finally, to practice being Ann Landers or someone like her and to write advice-giving letters to each other.

Cassette III

> **Side 1:** *Conflict-Resolution Model.* Dr. Harmin offers a formula for conflict resolution applicable in a wide variety of situations.
>
> **Side 2:** *A Girl and Her Dog.* What happens when we issue ultimatums and fail to communicate? And what would be the best thing for us to do if we were members of the family involved here?

Making Sense of Our Lives is available from Argus Communications, 7440 Natchez Avenue, Niles, Ill. 60648

Values Clarification with Sidney B. Simon. A series of reel tapes or cassettes in which Sidney Simon discusses some of his more popular strategies.

> **Side 1:** Introduction; here-and-now wheel; name tag with six values; introductory lecture on values in action; getting it together.
>
> **Side 2:** Forced choice game; "I learned" statements; five sentences for dirty arguing; "I resent" statements; "I demand" statements; "I appreciate" statements.
>
> **Side 3:** "Twenty things I love to do"; seven criteria for real values.
>
> **Side 4:** Simulation games; alligator river and fallout shelter; six sentences for communication; privacy blocks.
>
> **Side 5:** Practical considerations of values and behavior; alternative-search game; panel voting and rank ordering.
>
> **Side 6:** Panel (conclusion). The continuum; "I am proud" sentences; "I wonder" statements.

Values Clarification with Sidney B. Simon is available from the Espousal Center, 554 Lexington Street, Waltham, Mass. 02154

A REVIEW OF BOOKS IN VALUES CLARIFICATION[13]

Values clarification is one branch of the growing humanistic-education movement. The past decade has seen a proliferation of books on the topic. What follows is a review from a practitioner's point of view of some of the basic and major contributions to the field.

Raths, Louis; Harmin, Merrill; and Simon, Sidney B. *Values and Teaching*. Columbus, Ohio: Charles E. Merrill, 1966. 275 pp., $4.75.

[13]This review, by Joel Goodman, appeared in John E. Jones and William Pfeiffer's 1976 *Annual Handbook for Group Facilitators*. Iowa City, Iowa: University Associates, 1976.

This is the book that gave birth to the field. A major stimulus for the book was the increasing amount of values confusion experienced by young people. Bombarded by a myriad of influences (e.g. family, peer group, church, school, media) and enveloped in a world of accelerating change and future shock, many young people were/are experiencing confusion in such values-rich areas as love, sex, friendship, money, work, leisure, family, religion, and politics. The authors see this confusion reflected in such behavior patterns as apathy (listless, uninterested), flight (only fleeting interest), uncertainty (inability to make decisions), inconsistency (incompatible patterns in life), drifting (lack of enthusiasm and planning), overconforming (other-directed with a passion), overdissenting (chronic, irrational dissent), and posing (counterfeit role-playing).

Noting that traditional approaches to helping children develop values (e.g. setting an example, persuading and convincing, limiting choices, moralizing, inculcating, establishing rules, appealing to conscience) either do not work, or, in some cases, are inhumane, Raths and his associates have developed an approach which seeks to aid children in feeling valuable (positive, purposeful, enthusiastic, and proud). Thus, unlike many other educational books of the 60's, *Values and Teaching* goes beyond the diagnosis and offers a specific prescription. This is one of the book's (and the movement's) strengths: the values clarification theory has always had particular appeal in that it is complemented with many practical strategies. At the same time, the authors caution that "this value theory is not a panacea for all that ails children and education . . . [and] it does not pretend to help solve behavior difficulties whose causes lie outside of values issues" (p. 8).

The authors offer a valuing model based on the following definition of a value: (1) it must be chosen freely; (2) it must be chosen from among alternatives; (3) it must be chosen after thoughtful consideration of the consequences of each alternative; (4) it must be prized and cherished; (5) it must be something that one is willing to publicly affirm; (6) it must be acted upon; and (7) it must be done repeatedly, so as to be consistent with other life patterns. Something which does not meet *all* seven criteria is described as a value indicator (e.g. goals, purposes, aspirations, attitudes, interests, beliefs). Although values clarification has evolved in this area (see review of *Values Clarification: A Handbook of Practical Strategies for Teachers and Students*), these seven criteria provided the original foundation for the theory.

The authors operationalize this theory by presenting numerous practical strategies designed to help students examine their values against the background of the seven criteria. They devote two entire chapters to two basic and incredibly adaptable activities: the clarifying response and the values sheet. The clarifying response is at the heart of processing any values clarification exercise, while the values sheet is perhaps the easiest way to integrate subject matter and values exploration. The authors provide specific examples of each strategy, along with helpful guidelines for their use. Another chapter in the book introduces eighteen additional strategies.

Not only do the authors offer practical strategies, they also go on to provide support for the teacher just beginning to use values clarification. For example, in the chapter on "Getting Started: Guidelines and Problems," Raths, Harmin, and Simon respond to some common questions teachers ask.

Values and Teaching is a primer in the field of values clarification. Because of its background information and its helpful guidelines, as well as its description of some of the basic strategies, I heartily recommend this as a first book to pick up.

Simon, Sidney B.; Howe, Leland; and Kirschenbaum, Howard. *Values Clarification: A Handbook of Practical Strategies for Teachers and Students.* New York: Hart Publishing Co., 1972. 397 pp., $5.25.

Recipient of the Pi Lambda Theta "outstanding book" award, this volume has been acclaimed as the most useful collection of values clarification strategies yet published.

The authors begin with remarks on the values clarification approach and on ways to use this book. A significant element in this introduction is the move away from emphasizing the seven criteria of a value. Rather, the authors focus on the seven valuing skills or sub-processes (e.g. the ability to choose freely, the ability to consider alternatives and consequences). This change underlines the evolving process (as opposed to content) orientation of values clarification

The meat of this book is its smorgasbord of seventy-nine values clarification strategies. The strategies are presented in a very clear and sensible manner. "First comes the purpose, which always relates to one or more of the seven processes of valuing. Then the procedures are described in detail. Finally, there are notes and tips to the teacher, and additional suggestions if appropriate" (p. 22). These notes and tips often include helpful guidelines for processing the activity, brainstormed ways of adapting the procedure for different age levels, thoughts on sequencing, cautions (related to risk level) as well as numerous examples of the strategy (for example, there are 300 voting questions, over 260 public interview questions, 170 different rank orders, over 50 ideas for proudwhips, etc.).

The authors emphasize that there is no one right way to use a values clarification strategy. They encourage the reader to change and adapt the activities, as well as to think of new ones. This suggestion is crucial if the book is to avoid becoming a "cookbook crutch" that is followed blindly.

For those with experience in values clarification (through a workshop, course, or in-service program), this book can be a goldmine of "how to's." Hopefully, the reader will be able to hitchhike on these ideas and further expand the repertoire of valuing strategies.

Harmin, Merrill; Kirschenbaum, Howard; and Simon, Sidney B. *Clarifying Values Through Subject Matter.* Minneapolis: Winston Press, 1973. 146 pp., $3.25.

This easy-to-read book "offers one approach for making classrooms more relevant to a world of change, confusion, and conflict. It is not the only approach needed, but it is a practical one—something the teacher can use on Monday. Clarifying values through subject matter is a relatively simple method for the teacher to implement in his or her classroom; yet its implications are, we think, revolutionary" (p. 7).

This book is for the teacher who likes the values clarification approach, but wonders where to fit it in (considering that there is much pressure "to get to 1860" by the end of the semester). The authors propose a three-level teaching model, which suggests that almost any subject matter can be taught on three levels: factual, conceptual, values. The factual level involves the learning of specific information and basic skills (e.g. computational, penmanship). The conceptual level deals with abstractions, making generalizations from facts, examining cause and effect relationships. On the values level, students link the facts and concepts of a subject to their own lives. The authors stress that these three levels are interdependent (and not mutually exclusive, as some may assume).

As in their previous work, Harmin, Kirschenbaum, and Simon back up their theory with specific examples and practical suggestions. A major part of the book provides examples of three-level teaching in a wide variety of subject areas (ranging from the 3 R's to the fine arts to physical education to business courses to home economics to religion courses). The authors caution that they do not intend "to prescribe a curriculum in each subject. A few examples can hardly do justice to any subject area. But perhaps the examples will suggest a direction in which teachers in various disciplines may go" (p. 43).

In addition to planting seeds about three-level teaching, the authors also include a chapter by Clifford Knapp on using the values strategies with subject matter. Here, Knapp examines ways that fifteen strategies (drawn from *Values and Teaching* and *Values Clarification*) can be integrated within subject matter.

Perhaps the most provocative part of the book is a chapter entitled "Beyond the Third Level: What Is Worth Teaching?" The authors pose a series of values clarifying questions for the teacher: "Why am I teaching this subject area? Do I really believe my students need to have this knowledge or these skills? If I had no restraints or mandates imposed on me, what would I freely choose to teach? How does each area I am considering teaching relate to my students' lives? What are the real values dilemmas present in the subjects and themes I teach?" (p. 107). The authors proceed to enumerate several approaches to bridging the gap between subject matter and students' lives: the three-level approach, values units, values strategies, self-directed learning, and other humanistic approaches.

Harmin, Kirschenbaum, and Simon conclude with a three-level review of the book itself: They practice what they teach.

Kirschenbaum, Howard; and Simon, Sidney B., ed. *Readings in Values Clarification.* Minneapolis: Winston Press, 1973. 383 pp., $6.25.

Kirschenbaum and Simon have gathered here a good blend of conceptual and practical articles on values education. This comprehensive collection of thought-provoking readings is divided into six sections: "Values Clarification and Other Perspectives," "Values Clarification and School Subjects," "Values in Religious Education," "Values in the Family," "Other Applications for Values Clarification," and "An Annotated Bibliography."

The first section provides background on values clarification, paints the values education context in which it fits, examines the link between values clarification and futuristics, and draws on the expertise of others involved in values education (including Kohlberg, Rogers, and Rokeach) while exploring the cognitive-affective-active dimensions of valuing. The section closes with a very important, evolutionary article by Kirschenbaum: "Beyond Values Clarification." Here, he criticizes and expands on the original theory and suggests the need to integrate values clarification with other humanistic approaches to education.

"Values Clarification and School Subjects" is a good companion to *Clarifying Values Through Subject Matter.* This section includes twelve articles chock-full of ideas for three-level teaching and for using values strategies confluently.

There are an increasing number of religious educators who are excited about using values clarification. The third part of this book addresses that growing interest. Several articles speak to the need, the role, and the application of values clarification to religious education.

"Values in the Family" recognizes the great opportunity available to parents and children to learn from and with one another. This can all take place around the family dinner table, as illustrated in numerous examples of adaptations of values clarification strategies. The section ends with an article on listening skills, which are essential to any values clarification process—especially one involving different generations.

The fifth division in the book, "Other Applications for Values Clarification," is a stimulating potpourri of ways/people/places/times in which values clarification has been used. The authors punctuate the versatility of the approach by noting its use in such diverse settings and contexts as: a Black and Puerto Rican urban junior high school, a freshman dormitory at a rural university, in a national women's organization business meeting in Iowa, in Girl Scout programs nationwide, and in a large public school system-wide training program, among others.

This is a resource-full book. It closes with a resource-full annotated bibliography of articles and books that have been written on values clarification between 1965-1973. It leaves the reader with many next steps.

The four books reviewed above provide a solid foundation of readings in values clarification. In addition to these four, there are a number of publications which have added to the development of the field. These are annotated below.

Hawley, Robert; Simon, Sidney B.; and Britton, David. *Composition for Personal Growth: Values Clarification Through Writing.* New York: Hart Publishing Co., 1973. 184 pp., $5.25.

This teacher's handbook has a wealth of ideas on ways to develop writing skills and self-literacy simultaneously. The authors present many adaptable activities which aid students in "reading the book within themselves" and then in reflecting these values in composition and/or discussion. A number of schools are using this book in a confluent mode (integrated with a "traditional" English course) as well as congruently (as a course in itself).

Hawley, Robert, and Hawley, Isabel. *Human Values in the Classroom: A Handbook for Teachers.* New York: Hart Publishing Co., 1973. 320 pp., $4.95.

The Hawleys view human values as survival skills. In this book, they outline many specific teaching techniques and classroom procedures to enhance the development of valuing skills. Of particular help is the curriculum development sequence upon which they elaborate: orientation—community-building—achievement motivation—fostering open communication—information seeking, gathering, and sharing—value exploration and clarification—planning for change. The authors also focus on some issues of interest to these working on valuing in the classroom: grading and evaluation, approaches to discipline, creative problem-solving.

Hall, Brian P. *Value Clarification as Learning Process: A Guidebook.* New York: Paulist Press, 1973. 253 pp., $7.95.

As a companion guide to Hall's *Value Clarification as Learning Process: A Sourcebook* (in which value clarification theory is presented), this volume includes four sections: introduction, exercises in values clarification, conferences, and values strategies in the classroom. The author presents a number of strategies for students, teachers, and professionals through use of the following Pfeiffer and Jones-like format: introduction, materials needed, numbers, time, description of exercise, possible outcomes, application. The section on conferences outlines some alternative designs for introductory and advanced programs. Hall hopes that the reader will not blindly follow the strategy recipes and alternative workshop designs. Rather, he wants the book to "be a catalytic agent in helping those who wish to become involved in value clarification to create their own program" (p. 121).

Hawley, Robert. *Value Exploration Through Role-Playing.* New York: Hart Publishing Co., 1974. 176 pp., $4.95.

The author presents many helpful guidelines, formats, and examples of ways to use role-playing with junior and senior high school students. The book is spiced with numerous ideas for using role plays to focus on values and on decision-making skills. This is an excellent resource for teachers who are looking for the support and the know-how to use role-playing in the classroom.

Simon, Sidney B. *Meeting Yourself Halfway: Values Clarification for Daily Living.* Niles, Ill.: Argus, 1974. 102 pp., $5.25.

This is a catchy handbook/workbook that contains a month's worth of values clarification activities. Of the 31 activities, some are new and some are adaptations of ones appearing in *Values Clarification*. Dr. Simon has designed the strategies so that the reader can take a hands-on approach to this book—encouraging personal involvement and interaction with the material.

The above books are a sampling of some of the important contributions to the developing field of values clarification. In the future, we can expect new books to add to the depth and breadth of the field by focusing on such areas as: research in values clarification, applications of values clarification to specific areas of conflict and confusion (e.g. friendship, sexuality, consumerism, health), methodology for values curriculum development, and the development of facilitator skills.

ADDITIONAL READINGS TO GROW ON

Ashton-Warner, Sylvia. *Teacher*. New York: Bantam Books, 1963. A magnificent, personal story of an amazing woman and her inspiring method of teaching based on joy and love.

Borton, Terry. *Reach, Touch and Teach*. New York: McGraw-Hill Book Co., 1970. A readable, provacative, and informative introduction to process education for student concerns.

Brown, George Isaac. *Human Teaching for Human Learning*. New York: Viking Press, 1971. This book encompasses a philosophy and a process of teaching in which the affective or emotional aspects of learning flow together with the cognitive or intellectual functions.

Combs, Arthur, ed. *Perceiving, Behaving and Becoming*. Washington, D.C.: Association for Supervision and Curriculum Development, 1962. This book presents a series of articles by the leading educational theorists in perception, self-concept and self-actualization.

Fairfield, Roy P., ed. *Humanistic Frontiers in American Education*. Englewood Cliffs, N.J.: Prentice-Hall, Inc., 1971. This book offers new understanding of directions and goals, explores the forces shaping the future, and traces the birth of humanistic revolution to the impact John Dewey had upon education.

Fast, Julius. *Body Language*. New York: J. B. Lippincott Co. 1970. An entertaining survey of proxemics, kinesics, and nonverbal communication.

Greenberg, Herbert M. *Teaching with Feeling*. New York: Macmillan Publishing Co., 1969. This book focuses on the inner life of the teacher rather than the emotions of the learner. The author stresses "honesty, spontaneity and variety" in teaching.

Gunther, Bernard. *Sense Relaxation Below Your Mind*. New York: Collier Books, 1968. Gives exercises for individuals, partners, and groups to achieve greater sensory awareness. Many of the exercises are adaptable to class or group use.

Gunther, Bernard. *What to Do Till the Messiah Comes*. New York: Macmillan Publishing Co., 1971. This book demonstrates Gestalt therapy, group encounter, verbal and nonverbal ways to work through destructive behavior patterns and mind/body/energy blocks.

Gustaitis, Rasa. *Turning On*. New York: Macmillan Publishing Co., 1969. One woman's trip beyond LSD through awareness-expansion without the use of drugs. Included are discussion on truth-labs, gestalt therapy, meditation, Zen, sensory awareness, hip communes, brain-wave control.

Heath, Douglas H. *Humanizing Schools*. New York: Hayden Book Co., 1967. Through his analysis of a dropout's experience of personal estrangement, Heath develops a model of healthy maturing whereby he identifies the experiences young people need to become flexible, educable adults.

James, Muriel, and Jongeward, Dorothy. *Born to Win*. Reading, Mass.: Addison-Wesley Publishers, 1971. This book is primarily concerned with transactional analysis theory and its application to the daily life of the average person. Valuable to those in education, particularly the mental-health fields.

Jones, Richard M. *Fantasy and Feeling in Education*. New York: New York University Press, 1968. One of the few books in humanistic education written from the viewpoint of a Freudian-oriented psychoanalyst.

Lederman, Janet. *Anger and the Rocking Chair: Gestalt Awareness with Children*. New York: McGraw-Hill Book Co., 1969. This book is a dramatic, visual account of Gestalt methods with so-called "difficult" or "disturbed" children in elementary school.

Leonard, George B. *Education and Ecstasy*. New York: Delta Books, 1968. This book celebrates the joy, the unity, of learning and living—with practical suggestions on how to make this vision a reality in our schools.

Lowen, Alexander. *The Betrayal of the Body*. New York: Collier Books, 1967. This book charts a new course toward emotional fulfillment through body awareness and the recovery of a gratifying mind-body relationship.

Luft, Joseph. *Group Process*. Palo Alto, Calif.: National Press Books, 1970. Starting with the assumption that behavior is best understood in the context of interpersonal ties, the author establishes a basic framework within which components of the communication process may be viewed.

Lyon, Harold C. *Learning to Feel—Feeling to Learn*. Columbus, Ohio: Charles E. Merrill Publishing Co., 1971. A factual, down-to-earth book, giving straightforward accounts of the results experienced by the author as he tried out novel methods of bringing the "whole" student into the classroom, with the feeling aspects of himself, the intellectual aspects, and the capacity for self-responsibility.

Maslow, Abraham H. *Religions, Values, and Peak-Experiences*. New York: Viking Press, 1970. Maslow articulates on one of his prominent theses: the "religious" experience is a rightful subject for scientific investigation and speculation and, conversely, the "scientific community" will see its work enhanced by acknowledging and studying the specieswide need for spiritual expression which, in so many forms, is at the heart of "peak experiences" reached by healthy, fully functioning persons.

Montagu, Ashley. *Touching: The Human Significance of the Skin*. New York: Columbia University Press, 1971. Ashley Montagu presents a lively inquiry into the importance of tactile experience in the development of the person.

Nyberg, David. *Tough and Tender Learning.* Palo Alto, Calif.: National Press Books, 1971. A view of the current climate of the classroom and a method of approach the author feels would greatly improve the learning environment.

Otto, Herbert, and Mann, John. *Ways of Growth.* New York: Viking Press, 1968. This book brings together authoritative descriptions of contemporary methods of self-development. These efforts seek to cultivate normal human functioning beyond the level of average performance—in the matters of sensory awakening, sex, family, life, group living, and psychedelic experience.

Peterson, Severin. *A Catalog of the Ways People Grow.* New York: Ballantine Books, Inc., 1971. A catalog that presents description, excerpts from principal sources, and an extensive directory of information for the ways some people have found to grow.

Pfeiffer, William J., and Jones, John E. *Structured Experiences for Human Relations Training.* Iowa City, Iowa: University Associates Press, 1969-71. Each of three volumes contains detailed descriptions of about twenty-five "structured experiences," Some of the experiences are easily adaptable to the general classroom.

Purkey, William W. *Self Concept and School Achievement.* Englewood Cliffs, N.J.: Prentice-Hall, Inc., 1970. This book introduces an exciting new happening in contemporary education. This is the growing emphasis placed on the student's subjective and personal evaluation of himself as a dominant influence on his success or failure in school.

Rogers, Carl, and Stevens, Barry. *Person to Person.* Lafayette, Calif.: Real People Press, 1967. Professional papers by Rogers and others—about therapy, experiencing and learning—are set in a matrix of personal response and the use that Barry Stevens has made of these papers arriving at better understanding of herself, and her view of the problem of being human as she encountered it in her life.

Rubin, Theodore Isaac. *The Angry Book.* New York: Macmillan Publishing Co., 1969. An easy-to-read essay encouraging readers to allow themselves to be constructively angry.

Ruitenbeek, Hendrik M. *The New Group Therapies.* New York: Discus Books, 1970. A guide to the dynamic effectiveness of the human growth potential experience.

Spolin, Viola. *Improvisation for the Theater.* Evanston, Ill.: Northwestern University Press, 1963. The book describes about two hundred games that have been played with children and teens learning to act, games that involve emotional expression, sensory awareness, and a sense of place. The ideas are easily adaptable to personal-relations work and are fun.

Thelen, Herbert A. *Education and the Human Quest.* Chicago: University of Chicago Press, 1972. The author presents four learning experiences that he believes a child must have to become educated—personal inquiry, group investigation, reflection, and skill development.

Weinstein, Gerald, and Fantini, Mario D. *Toward Humanistic Education.* New York: Praeger Publishers, 1970. Based on a model that engages the child as a whole-hearted participant in the educational process by making that process "relevant" to him in the most profound sense.

NATIONAL HUMANISTIC EDUCATION CENTER

Materials Available on Values Clarification

1. **Values and Teaching** by Louis Raths, Merrill Harmin & Sidney B. Simon. (Columbus, Ohio: Charles E. Merrill, 1966). The basic text on the "values clarification approach."

2. **Values Clarification: A Handbook of Practical Strategies for Teachers and Students** by Sidney Simon, Leland Howe & Howard Kirschenbaum (New York: Hart Publishing, 1972). Seventy-nine methods for values clarification are described, with instructions for the teacher and numerous examples of the basic strategies.

3. **Clarifying Values Through Subject Matter** by Merrill Harmin, Howard Kirschenbaum & Sidney B. Simon (Minneapolis, Winston Press, 1973). A three-level theory of subject matter and examples of how every subject in the curriculum can be taught with a focus on values.

4. **Readings in Values Clarification** edited by Howard Kirschenbaum and Sidney Simon (Minneapolis: Winston, Press, 1973). Includes most of the articles below, plus essays by Kohlberg, Rokeach, Rogers, Holt, Bronfenbrenner, Kirschenbaum, Simon and others.

5. **Personalizing Education: Values Clarification and Beyond** by Leland and Mary Martha Howe (Hart, 1975). 100 new ideas and strategies built into a framework for sequencing v. c. activities.

6. **Composition for Personal Growth: Values Clarification Through Writing** by Sidney Simon, Robert Hawley & David Britton (New York: Hart Publishing, 1973).

7. **Values in Sexuality** by Eleanor Morrison & Mila Underhill Price (New York: Hart Publishing, 1974). Values clarification strategies with a focus on human sexuality education.

8. **Making Sense of Our Lives** by Merrill Harmin (Niles, IL: Argus, 1973). Two dozen lessons on values and communication for pre-teens through adults. You receive a package containing 24 color posters to motivate each lesson, 24 ditto masters to produce student activity sheets, and teacher instructions.

9. **Meeting Yourself Halfway: Values Clarification for Daily Living** by Sidney Simon (Niles, IL: Argus, 1974). V.C. for personal growth.

10. **Values in Teaching** by Sidney Simon. Two cassette tapes.

11. **Value Cassettes** by Merrill Harmin (Argus, 1974). Three tapes, each with two value clarifying experiences, teacher directions, and spirit masters for student worksheets. Age 10 thru adults.

12. An Annotated Bibliography on Values Clarification by Kirschenbaum, Glaser & Gray.

13. **Songs From Values Workshops** about 20 popular songs, recorded and published by Marianne Simon. Cassette tape.

14. "Current Research in Values Clarification" by Kirschenbaum (Sept. 1975).

15. "How Can We Teach Values?" a three article pamphlet containing "Three Ways to Teach Church School" and "Your Values Are Showing" by Sidney Simon and "How Can We Teach Values?" by John Westerhoff

16. "Values Clarification at the Family Table" by Kirschenbaum and "Dinner Table Learning" by Simon. Two related articles in one pamphlet

17. "Teaching Environmental Education with a Focus on Values" by Clifford Knapp. Many good exercises and activities.

18. "In Defense of Values Clarification" by Kirschenbaum. Harmin, Howe & Simon. A position paper and response to some criticisms

Numbers 19-27 are article reprints

19. "Teaching English with a Focus on Values" by Kirschenbaum and Simon.
20. "Teaching History with A Focus on Values" by Harmin, Simon and Kirschenbaum.
21. "Teaching Afro-American History with a Focus on Values" by Simon and Carnes.
22. "Teaching Science with a Focus on Values" by Harmin, Kirschenbaum and Simon.
23. "Teaching Health Education with a Focus on Values" by Betof and Kirschenbaum.
24. "The Search for Values with a Focus on Math" by Harmin, Kirschenbaum and Simon.
25. "Teaching Home Economics with a Focus on Values" by Kirschenbaum.
26. "Values Clarification vs. Indoctrination" by Simon (theory).
27. "Values" by Harmin and Simon (theory and bibliography).

Materials Available on Humanistic Education

28. **Freedom to Learn** by Carl Rogers (Columbus, Ohio: Charles E. Merrill, 1969). A basic text in humanistic education.

29. **Humanistic Education Sourcebook** edited by Don Read & Sidney Simon (Prentice-Hall, 1975). Readings by major figures in the humanistic education movement

30. **WAD-JA-GET? The Grading Game in American Education** by Howard Kirschenbaum, Sidney Simon & Rodney Napier (NY: Hart Publishing, 1971). Pros, cons, history, research, alternatives—built into an easy to read novel.

31. **Understanding the Problem Child** by Louis Raths & Anna Burrell (Danville, NJ: Economics Press, 1963). Title should be "Understanding People." Has 200 suggestions to help teachers meet the emotional needs of students. (This pamphlet is the foundation of "IALAC")

32. **People Projects** by Merrill Harmin. (Addison-Wesley, 1974). Colorful task cards, with a V.C. humanistic focus. 40 cards per set. Set A (ages 9-11), Set B (ages 10-12), Set C (ages 11-13).

33. **Process Posters** by Merrill Harmin (Argus, 1974). Fifteen large, illustrated posters, each outlining a humanistic process: I Learneds, Conflict Resolution Model, Support Group Tasks, etc.

34. "What We Know About Learning" by Arthur Combs. A cassette tape. The implications of humanistic psychological theory and research for teaching, learning and evaluation.

35. **The Human Side of Human Beings** by Harvey Jackins (Rational Island, 1965). The theory of re-evaluation counseling, a good, psychological foundation for humanistic education.

HUMANISTIC EDUCATORS NETWORK

36. A yearly membership brings you periodic mailings with **Articles, Resources, Teaching Ideas** and other information on humanistic education. These are printed on 3-holed, notebook sized paper, enabling members to build their own cumulative notebook on humanistic education.

37. "IALAC" by Sidney Simon. The famous story, antidote to the killer statement, in an attractive pamphlet, with suggestions for classroom use

38. "Humanisticography" by John Canfield & Mark Phillips. An annotated resource guide to over 130 books, films, tapes, simulations, classroom exercise books, curricula, journals & organizations in the field of humanistic education.

Numbers 35-42 are article reprints.

39. "What Is Humanistic Education?" by Kirschenbaum.
40. "Can We Humanize Foreign Language Education" by Wattenmaker & Wilson.
41. "What Is a Good School?" by Neil Postman.
42. "The Listening Game" by Kirschenbaum. Communication exercises
43. "Sensitivity Modules" by Kirschenbaum & Simon. Activites.
44. For a listing of other materials on humanistic education, ask for NHEC's current brochure.

For additional information, write to:
NATIONAL HUMANISTIC EDUCATION CENTER
110 Spring Street
Saratoga Springs, New York 12866

INDEX

Active listening (focusing), 147
Active skills, 16, 143
Affective education, 148
Affective skills, 16, 143
Alone time, 148
Alschuler, Alfred, 125

Berger, Bonnie, 22
Berman, Louise, 11
Birth control information, 3
Blokker, William, 23
Borton, Terry, 14
Brainstorming, 148
Britton, David, 175

Cassettes, in values clarification, 169-170
Clarifying responses, 24-26, 142
Clarifying Values Through Subject Matter (Harmin, Kirschenbaum and Simon), 9, 28, 173-174
Closure, 148
Coat-of-arms activity, 133-134
Cognitive skills, 15, 143
Cole, Henry, 11-12

Composition for Personal Growth (Hawley, Simon and Britton), 175
Conroy, Gladys, 22
Continua, 27, 131-132

Dear Me letter, 127-128
Dear Teacher letter, 135
Death, 21, 32-33
Defuzzing wheel, 128-130
Devaluation, 14-15
Dewey, John, 8
Diary, 87-88
Drug education, values clarification activities and, 60-73
  inventory, 71-72
  moral dilemmas, 69
  rank-ordering, 60-63
  spread of opinion, 67
  values-voting, 65
  writing strategies, 95-97

Ecology, 21, 30, 32
Emergency Now exercise, 113-120
Environment, 21, 30, 32

184 INDEX

Evaluation, 121-138
  coat of arms, 133-134
  continuum, 131-132
  Dear Me letter, 127-128
  Dear Teacher letter, 135
  defuzzing wheel, 128-130
  feedforward form, 126
  guidelines for humanistic, 122-125
  New and Good Calendar, 136
  Nice Things Box, 136-137
  observation, 134-135
  rank-ordering, 130-131
  standardized instruments, 135-136
  voting questions, 132
  whatcha know, whatcha need to know, 130
Eurich, Alvin, 33

Facilitator, 149
Family life, 19, 21
Fantasy, 149
Fantini, Mario D., 3
Feedback, 125, 143, 149
Feedforward, 143
Feedforward form, 126
Films, in values clarification, 166-169
Future Shock (Toffler), 12

Glasser, William, 3
Goodlad, John, 121
Goodman, Joel, 22, 23
Grading, 122-123, 143
Greenberg, Jerrold S., 23
Growing old, 21

Hall, Brian P., 176
Harmin, Merrill, 9, 11, 22, 25, 28, 170-174
Hawkins, Laurie, 22
Hawley, Isabel, 175
Hawley, Robert, 175, 176
Hopp, Joyce W., 23
Hopp, Norma Joyce, 22, 23
Howe, Leland, 9, 172-173
Human sexuality, values clarification
    activities and, 40-59
  inventory, 55-59
  moral dilemmas, 50-53
  rank-ordering, 40-43
  spread of opinion, 48-49
  values-voting, 45-46
  writing strategies, 88-95

Human Values in the Classroom: A Handbook for Teachers (Hawley and Hawley), 175

I learned (relearned) statements, 149
Icebreaker activity, 108, 110, 112
Interpersonal skills, 16, 143
Inventory, 27, 35, 39
  defined, 150
  drug education and, 71-72
  human sexuality and, 55-59
  nutrition education and, 84
Ivey, Allen, 125

Jourard, Sidney, M., 153

Kelley, Paul, 22
Killer statements, 103, 150
Kirschenbaum, Howard, 9, 15, 22, 28, 172-175
Knapp, Clifford E., 10, 22

Maslow, Abraham, 87
Meeting Yourself Halfway: Values Clarification for Daily Living (Simon), 176
Modlin, Herbert C., 3
Monsour, Karem J., 3
Moral dilemmas, 27, 35, 39
  drug education and, 69
  human sexuality and, 50-53
  nutrition education and, 80
Moreno, J. L., 152
Morrison, Eleanor, 23
Munson, Howard E., 23

Name tags, 108, 110, 112
National Humanistic Education Center (NHEC), 9, 138, 145
Negotiating, 150
New and Good Calendar activity, 136
Nice Things Box, 136-137
Nutrition education, values clarification
    activities and, 74-75
  inventory, 84
  moral dilemmas, 80
  rank-ordering, 74-76
  spread of opinion, 82
  values-voting, 78-79
  writing strategies, 98-99

INDEX

Observation, 134-135
Osman, Jack D., 22

Page, David, 21
Parris, Cynthia, 23
Peanuts, 13, 15
Peer-group pressure, 150
Personal diary, 87-88
Planning for exercise, 102
Positive focus, 151
Positive strokes, 151
Positive teacher-modeling, 154
Postman, Neil, 149
Processing
   Emergency Now exercise, 113-120
   icebreaker activity, 108, 110, 112
   name tags, 108, 110, 112
   stages in, 105
   types of, 151-152

Raettig, Vilma, 22
Rank-ordering, 27, 35, 38
   drug education and, 60-63
   evaluation and, 130-131
   human sexuality and, 40-43
   nutrition education and, 74-76
Raths, Louis E., 8-9, 10, 11, 21, 25, 170-172
Read, Donald A., 23
Readings in Values Clarification (Kirschenbaum and Simon), 9, 174-175
Rees, Floyd D., 22, 23
Responsibility for oneself, 154-155
Risk-taking, 152
Rogers, Carl, 5, 11
Role-playing, 152

Safety, 21
Self-concept, 153
Self-disclosure, 153
Self-evaluation, 153
Self-identity, 3
Sexuality, *see* Human sexuality
Sharing, 153
Significant others, 153
Simon, Sidney B., 9, 11, 22, 23, 25, 28, 170-176
Spread of opinion, 35, 38-39
   drug education and, 67
   human sexuality and, 48-49
   nutrition education and, 82

Strategy, defined, 153-154
Support groups, 154

Tapes, in values clarification, 169-170
Terminology, 147-155
Three-level teaching/learning, 27-33, 142
Toffler, Alvin, 12
Trust, 154

Underhill, Mila, 23

Value Clarification as Learning Process: A Guidebook (Hall), 176
Value Clarification as Learning Process: A Sourcebook (Hall), 176
Value Exploration Through Role-Playing (Hawley), 176
Values, 7-8
Values clarification
   activities, *see* Values clarification activities
   adaptability of, 28
   clarifying responses, 24-26, 142
   definition of, 16
   films in, 166-169
   flexibility of, 23-24
   need for, 10-15
   review of books, 22-23, 170-180
   tapes and cassettes in, 169-170
   three-level teaching/learning, 27-33, 142
   values sheets, 27, 28-29, 156-166
Values Clarification: A Handbook of Practical Strategies for Teachers and Students (Simon, Howe and Kirschenbaum), 9, 172-173
Values clarification activities, 26-27, 35-85, 143
   context of, 36-37
   directions for, 37-39
   inventory, 27, 35, 39
      drug education and, 71-72
      human sexuality and, 55-59
      nutrition education and, 84
   moral dilemmas, 27, 35, 39
      drug education and, 69
      human sexuality and, 50-53
      nutrition education and, 80
   processing, 102, 105-120
      Emergency Now exercise, 113-120
      icebreaker activity, 108, 110, 112
      name tags, 108, 110, 112
      stages in, 105

Values clarification activities (cont.)
  purpose of, 36
  rank-ordering, 27, 35, 38
    drug education and, 60-63
    human sexuality and, 40-43
    nutrition education and, 74-76
  spread of opinion, 35, 38-39
    drug education and, 67
    human sexuality and, 48-49
    nutrition education and, 82
  values-voting, 27, 35, 38
    drug education and, 65
    human sexuality and, 45-46
    nutrition education and, 78-79
  writing strategies, 87-99
    drug education and, 95-97
    human sexuality and, 88-95
    nutrition education and, 98-99
Values sheets, 27, 28-29, 156-166

Values and Teaching (Raths, Harmin and Simon), 9, 170-172
Values-voting, 27, 35, 38
  drug education and, 65
  evaluation and, 132
  human sexuality and, 45-46
  nutrition education and, 78-79
Voting questions, *see* Values-voting

Walker, Marie Hartwell, 23
Weingartner, Charles, 149
Weinstein, Gerald, 3
Whatcha know, whatcha need to know exercise, 130
Wilgoren, Richard, 11
Writing strategies, 87-89
  drug education and, 95-97
  human sexuality and, 88-95
  nutrition education and, 98-99